The Power of Presence

THE POWER OF PRESENCE

PRESENCE

A love story

NEIL T. ANDERSON

MONARCH
BOOKS

Oxford, UK, and Grand Rapids, USA

Published by Monarch Books
an imprint of
Lion Hudson plc
Wilkinson House, Jordan Hill Road,
Oxford OX2 8DR, England
Email: monarch@lionhudson.com
www.lionhudson.com/monarch

ISBN 978 0 85721 731 8
e-ISBN 978 0 85721 732 5

First edition 2016

Acknowledgments
Scripture quotations taken from are from The Holy Bible, English Standard Version® (ESV®) copyright © 2001 by Crossway, a publishing ministry of Good News Publishers. All rights reserved.

A catalogue record for this book is available from the British Library

Printed and bound in the UK, March 2016, LH26

Contents

FOREWORD   7

ACKNOWLEDGMENTS   11

INTRODUCTION   13

CHAPTER 1: THE ABSENCE OF
PRESENCE   19

CHAPTER 2: SUFFERING IN
HIS PRESENCE   33

CHAPTER 3: COMING INTO HIS
PRESENCE   53

CHAPTER 4: MINISTERING IN HIS
PRESENCE   71

CHAPTER 5: RESTING IN HIS
PRESENCE   93

CHAPTER 6: FULLY IN HIS PRESENCE   115

FURTHER RESOURCES   135

Foreword

If you were a renowned author whose books had been read by millions; if you had founded a successful Christian ministry and had the large conferences, films, publishing deals, and international travel that go with that; if you had seen God work through you to radically transform countless lives... would you be prepared to give it all up if God said so? And if you did give it up, can you imagine that you could possibly be happy with the turn your life had taken?

I have had the immense privilege of being friends with Neil and Joanne Anderson for the best part of twenty years. I have observed at close quarters how Joanne, a feisty lady of enormous intelligence and humor with an incredible gift for godly discernment, succumbed to dementia. And how Neil – without a second thought – dropped everything to care for her and, more importantly, to *be* with her.

This small volume is a beautiful love story that will move you deeply. You will enter into the story of Neil and Joanne Anderson and their life together. But beyond that you will see the story of your life and your ministry in a new light. You will gain a deeper appreciation of the relationship that your Creator and Savior longs to have with you, and realize afresh that He does not intend your life to be primarily about *doing* but about *being*.

I am so grateful to God for the message that He has given to the church through Neil and Joanne: that *every* Christian can take hold of their freedom in Christ and become a fruitful disciple of Jesus. As I lead Freedom in Christ Ministries, the ministry they founded, and see Neil spending day after day out of the limelight simply *being* with Joanne and yet genuinely content and more in love with her than ever, I see someone who is living out the message God gave him.

If you are in Christian ministry, I urge you to read this book. It will only take a couple of hours but the effect could last a lifetime as it helps you reevaluate the balance between *being* and *doing*.

If you find yourself in difficult life circumstances – especially, perhaps, if you too are caring for a loved one – this book will help you find comfort and rediscover the incredible purpose God has called you to.

And if you simply want to learn how to know Jesus better, you will not be disappointed.

Steve Goss
Executive Director
Freedom in Christ Ministries International

Acknowledgments

I want to thank Tony Collins for being a friend of Freedom in Christ Ministries. Tony has a storied career in Christian publishing and, sadly for us, is retiring. Publishing is a big industry, and associations with authors and ministry can be little more than business. With Tony it was friendship and ministry, while still being a good businessman. He also helped me and others to be better writers. Here is to you, Tony. May you have a well-deserved retirement, and many happy years of choosing the jobs you want to do, but don't feel you have to do.

Introduction

"Earth to Neil! Earth to Neil! You're out in your garden again." I always wondered how she knew when I was present in body, but absent in spirit. Joanne was frustratingly accurate in her discernment when my mind was somewhere else. Many were the nights when I heard from the other half of the bed we shared for nearly fifty years, "Turn off your brain, Anderson!" How did she know that I was rewriting a chapter in one of my books? She is the most discerning person I know, which has proven invaluable for the kind of ministry God has called us to.

Now I'm sitting in silence in a skilled nursing/long-term care facility. Agitated dementia has been slowly eating away Joanne's brain, which makes it hard for her sensitive mind to function well. She read two to three books a week for many years, but now she can't remember what medicine she took ten minutes ago. I suspended all international travel three years ago so we could have some time together. Ministry had dominated our life for most of those fifty years, which prompted her to ask, "When is it *our* time?"

Our time turned out to be very different from what we planned, but not what God planned.

She seldom asks about our children or grandchildren, whom she loved. She doesn't want any visitors, except me. The only thing that brightens her day is when I walk into her private room, which I do at least twice daily. As I walk through the door, and before she sees me, I say, "Beep! Beep!" Instantly, she knows it's me, and says, "Oh Daddy." Only in the last six months has she called me "Daddy," and there is only one human being on this planet that can fulfill that need for her.

We don't talk much, because it takes too much energy. I have become keenly aware that God is using Joanne's illness to teach me about the power of presence. I'm learning on a much deeper level the purpose of just being there, and what it means to be still and know that He is God. Being alone with my soulmate, best friend, and lover is not a "come down" for one who has traveled the world. It has been a "come up." There is an inexplicable peace that comes from knowing I don't have to *do* in order to *be* in God's will – to be in His presence – to be in each other's presence.

Many have noted that the caregiver of one suffering from dementia or Alzheimer's disease is the one who actually suffers the most. For the first two and a half years I took care of Joanne at home. Doing so is a twenty-four-hour, seven-day-a-week job that progressively gets more difficult. It is like raising a child who is regressing rather than maturing. Instead of potty training, one has to cope with incontinence. She has always been such a modest lady; I desperately wanted to spare her from all the indignities that come from the loss of control, but I couldn't. At the skilled nursing facility she strongly prefers that I do her bathing and grooming, which I do. I know it sounds strange, but that is our time together. It's my presence she longs for. She has my full attention. There are no more "earth to Neils."

In our "retirement" there have been no day trips, vacations, movies, or dining out. It sounds bleak, but in all honesty I can say that it hasn't been. In fact, it has been a peaceful time of reflection upon the presence of God, and how that has shaped me, our marriage, and ministry. My theology tells me that God is omnipresent; however, we are not always aware of His presence, and yet without His presence we are not fully alive.

What we call socials or fellowship usually falls far short of the spiritual union implied in *koinonia*. A civil union between two people is not the same as a marriage where two become one in Christ. Most celebrants at the Lord's Table are falling far short of the communion God wants to have with His children. In fact, words cannot capture the essence of what it means to be fully in communion with God and others. It is not a location or an activity. It is a state of being – a mingling together of one another's presence.

This is not a book about dementia or Alzheimer's disease. It is a reflection on the presence of God, and what it means to be in His presence during the loneliest and most difficult times of our lives. I will share some of Joanne's struggles with dementia, because that is the context in which I am presently experiencing what I am writing about. My silent times with Joanne have given me the opportunity to reflect on over forty-five years of pastoral work, and recount how God's presence has transformed me and shaped a global ministry.

Chapter One is about the absence of presence, and the fear of being alone or abandoned. From the beginning God has said it isn't good for us to be alone. We absolutely need God, and we necessarily need each other. Imagine being totally alone in the presence of evil, and how frightening that would be. Why did the Old Testament make no distinction between death and hell, using the same word for both?

Chapter Two deals with suffering in the presence of God. What do we do in hard times when God seems to be absent, when He suspends His conscious blessings? Twice before, God has taken Joanne and me through dark times that brought about monumental changes in our lives for the good. Now we are experiencing His ministry of darkness again, but this time it is different.

Chapter Three is about coming into His presence. What does it mean to pray by the Spirit? How does prayer become two-way instead of one-way? There is no dialogue when only one is present. Every believer is hearing from God, but many are unaware of it. How should we come into His presence? What good is prayer if God isn't present?

Chapter Four covers ministering in God's presence. How many activities in the name of "ministry" would continue as scheduled if the Holy Spirit were absent? How does the omnipresence of God enter into our ministry? Does He work alone, or do we work together? What is God's role in ministry and what is ours? Can we even call it ministry if God's persence isn't an integral part of it? Didn't Jesus say that apart from Him we can do nothing?

Chapter Five is about resting in His presence. God told Moses that His presence would go with him and He would give him rest. How does His presence go with us, and how does forty years of wandering in the wilderness constitute rest? Jesus said, "Come to me and I will give you rest." What is the sabbath rest that remains? How do we enter into His rest?

The final chapter considers what it means to be fully in His presence. Someday we shall see Him face to face. Oh, what a glorious day that will be! What will it be like to be in the presence of eternal goodness with a complete absence of evil? We can't even fathom that. We can only hope and long for it, but until then we can learn to practice His presence now. My prayer is that this little book will cause you to "seek his presence continually" (Psalm 105:4).

Neil T. Anderson

1

The Absence of Presence

In taking upon Himself a human soul, He also took upon Himself the affections of the soul. As God He was not distressed, but as a human He was capable of being distressed. It was not as God He died, but as man. It was in human voice that He cried: "My God, My God, why have You forsaken Me?" As human, therefore, He speaks on the cross, bearing with Him our terrors. For amid dangers it is a very human response to think ourself abandoned. As human, therefore, He is distressed, weeps, and is crucified.

Ambrose

Every night I help Joanne do her "ablutions." That is what she called her evening bathroom rituals, which always seemed to take an inordinate amount of time. I thought that "ablutions" was a word she made up to describe her routine. I was surprised to find out that "ablution" is a real word that means a washing or cleansing of the body. Being a prolific reader, her vocabulary is more extensive than mine. Her degree is in home economics and food, but it should have been English literature. She typed all my papers, two master's theses, and a doctoral dissertation for my first four degrees. When Biola University supplied all the faculty with an Apple computer, I knew I needed to learn how to type. Joanne taught me how, and I typed my final dissertation and every book since. She was also the first editor of all my books. What a blessing that has been to me. She corrected more than my grammar. She provided a feminine critique of our message. I say "our" because we have lived our message together. Her name only appears on two of my books, *Daily in Christ* and *Overcoming Depression*, but there is a little of her presence in every book.

After she finishes dinner at night I help her to the bathroom. She sits in front of the sink and asks, "What do I do next?" Even simple routines have become cloudy. I wash her face and put on the night cream that has kept her looking much younger than she is. She is a physical wreck, but Joanne has the skin of a twenty-year-old. I bought her a power toothbrush that she motors around her mouth, while remnants of her evening meal come drooling out. People with dementia have trouble swallowing, and food stays in their mouth like a chipmunk. Then it's off to bed.

I used to pray for her before I left every night, but for the last few months she has been praying: "Now I lay me down to sleep. I pray the Lord my soul to keep. If I should die before I wake, I pray the Lord my soul to take." Then she says the Lord's Prayer. Short-term memory is gone, but remnants of long-term memory linger. She is like a little girl saying a child's prayer, but the sincerity in which it is said brings tears to my eyes. The Lord is still in residence.

I often stay until she is asleep. One evening I had drifted off to sleep myself when she suddenly broke the silence with a desperate cry of "Neil!"

It startled me. I said, "I'm here, Babe."

"Oh, I was afraid you were gone," she replied. She had been mentioning some struggles with fear, which puzzled me at first. We had talked many times in the past about fear. She once had a fear of flying, but overcame that and was able to travel with me when she wanted. She also edited *Freedom from Fear*, which I wrote with Rich Miller. So she has an above average understanding of what constitutes the God-given ability to fear the objects that threaten our physical and psychological safety, and could normally distinguish that from an irrational fear or phobia. She also knew that physical death is no longer a legitimate fear object. Paul said, "For to me to live is Christ, and to die is gain" (Philippians 1:21). So what was she afraid of?

A similar cry came from the middle cross two thousand years ago. "And at the ninth hour Jesus cried out with a loud voice, 'Eloi, Eloi, lema sabachthani?' which means, 'My God, my God, why have you forsaken me?'" (Mark 15:34). Nietzche said, "God is dead, and we have killed him." Such apostasy overlooks one of the most basic tenets of Christianity. Jesus was fully human *and* fully God. He was one person, with two natures. God didn't die, but the One who came in the flesh did physically die. The concept of being alive means *to be in union with*, and to die means *to be separated from*. We are physically alive when our souls are in union with our bodies, and we are spiritually alive when our souls are in union with God. That is why the early church defined salvation as union with God. Like Adam, Jesus was both physically and spiritually alive. Unlike Adam He never sinned, and therefore never died spiritually, even though He was tempted in every way that we are. From the middle cross also came these words, "Father, into your hands I commit my spirit" (Luke 23:46).

The Apostles' Creed states that Jesus descended into *hell*, which is the Hebrew word *sheol*. Hebrew has only one word for hell and death, and that is *sheol* (in Greek, *hades*). The emphasis is on separation, not destination. It was the separation of His human nature from the Father that caused Him to cry out. Between the excruciating pain of the crucifixion and the resurrection, Jesus took the plunge into the abyss of aloneness – complete abandonment – which is a frightening prospect.

The fear that comes from being totally alone speaks to our vulnerability. We cannot rationally explain it away. That is what Joanne sensed that evening. Almost every time I leave the room Joanne asks if I will be back that evening or the next morning. If she doesn't ask, I tell her that I will always be there for her, and I mean it. So does God. He says, "I will never leave you nor forsake you" (Hebrews 13:5), which qualifies Him to say, "Fear not. I am present with you in your distress, whether you sense My presence or not."

In that moment of separation Jesus quotes from Psalm 22. His cry of agony is a prayer: "My God, My God." While the mocking crowd and the first thief have given up their faith in God, Jesus clings to it. What an incredible example that is for us in the hour of our greatest despair. In the midst of His own abandonment, He declares the nearness of God.

In the beginning of time God said that it was not good for us to be alone. Imagine how you would feel if you were in a mortuary and entered a room alone where the corpse of a stranger was displayed? Would you feel uneasy? Eerie? Maybe you would feel a little frightened even though you know that the dead person can do you no harm? This is not the fear of anything in particular, but the fear of being alone with death. This speaks to the most basic of human needs – to have a sense of belonging – and why many struggle with issues of abandonment.

Such a fear cannot be overcome by a rational explanation of its groundlessness. A child's fear of walking through the woods alone on a dark night can only be overcome by the presence of another. The uneasiness of sitting alone with a corpse disappears when a friend or family member joins you in the room.

When I was a young child on the farm I woke up one afternoon from a nap. I went downstairs but didn't see anybody. "Mom, where are you?" I asked. There was no answer. It was a warm summer day, so I assumed that my parents and siblings were outside. I ventured out with the hope of finding someone, but they were nowhere to be found. The apprehension mounted as I raced from the barn to the cornfields. I was almost overcome with fear, but it was immediately eradicated upon seeing the family car turn into the quarter-mile-long lane that led to our house. They had taken a quick run to a neighboring farm thinking that they would be back before I woke up.

I was pedaling a stationary bike, rehabbing my knee and watching television, when I saw another plane hit the second tower of the World Trade Center on September 11, 2001. Instantly, I knew it was no accident. Even though Joanne was home with me I felt an urgent need to be with other people. I just needed to be a part of our collective humanity, which had just been assaulted. I wanted to be in the presence of others and share in our common grief. I really don't have adequate words to describe the power of presence. I just know that it is real, and without it we suffer.

A similar reaction happened when Islamist terrorists attacked and killed two police officers and the staff of the satirical publication *Charlie Hebdo*, in January 2015. To protest the atrocity, forty world leaders joined hands in solidarity with 3.7

million people. It was the largest demonstration in France's history. Some of those world leaders were sworn enemies of each other, but they set aside their differences for a day to stand together against a greater threat to all humanity. Sadly, there was no significant presence from the US executive branch of government. They missed an opportunity to say to the rest of the free world, "We're with you, and we are in this together."

Our presence or absence at certain events speaks volumes to others. When my children were growing up I always made a point of circling important dates in my calendar that involved my immediate family. I don't think I ever missed one of Karl's soccer or baseball games. If someone asked for an appointment to see me when I was a pastor, I would tell them I was already booked for that time unless it was a catastrophic event. I felt no guilt or obligation to tell them that I was already committed to be with my family. My secretary couldn't tell my wife or children that I was unavailable if they called. She could say that I was with someone, and give them the choice of whether it was right to interrupt what I was doing. Family members feel abandoned when a spouse or parent is not there for them in times of need. I almost never traveled for ministry when my children were still living at home. If I did, I tried to take them with me. Many family vacations were intertwined with ministry. Usually that was the only way we could afford a vacation.

The quality of presence is determined by our capacity to love. "There is no fear in love, but perfect love casts out fear" (1 John 4:18). Imagine being raised in a family where there is no love shown to one another. It would be a house full of people who are all alone. A living hell. Many years ago, a shy college student shared that her mother had remarried a man whom she feared. She, in turn, totally rejected him as the head of their "home." In retaliation he forbade her to eat with the rest of the family. So she ate her meals alone in her bedroom. They hadn't spoken one word to each other in two years. She professed to be a believer, but her stepfather wasn't.

I asked her if she loved him.

"No," she said. "I hate him."

"Do you want to go on living like this?" I asked.

Of course she didn't, but she didn't know what to do about it. So we worked out a plan. That night she was to go home and ask his permission to talk to him. If he granted her that permission, she was going to ask his forgiveness for not loving him and not accepting him as the head of their home.

She followed through on that commitment, and he said, "My God, I have a daughter."

Hell is loneliness where no love can penetrate. It is the total absence of God, who is love. In the final judgment those whose names are not written in the Lamb's Book of Life will be cast out of His presence. That is hell. Heaven is to be completely in His presence. Experiencing His presence now is a taste of heaven on earth. It is understandable why the Old Testament has only one word for hell and death, because they are essentially the same.

In contrast, I have been in the presence of evil that defies description. It is not a time when you want to be alone, because fear can immediately engulf you. There is no rational reason why we should be afraid if we know the truth, because Satan is disarmed. However, did reading that last sentence, which is absolutely true, wipe away all your fears about a possible future encounter with a demonic spirit? Would you feel better if I was there with you at the time? Sorry, but I can't be there for you. Would you feel better if Almighty God was present with you in the same room at the same time? He is.

It should surprise no one that most spiritual attacks happen when we are alone, and mostly at night. One of Job's friends had such an encounter (Job 4:12–17):

Now a word was brought to me stealthily; my ear received the whisper of it. Amid thoughts from visions of the night, when deep sleep falls on men, dread came upon me, and trembling, which made all my bones shake. A spirit glided past my face; the hair of my flesh stood up. It stood still, but I could not discern its appearance. A form was before my eyes; there was silence, then I heard a voice: "Can mortal man be in the right before God? Can a man be pure before his Maker?"

"A word" was not "a word from the Lord." God doesn't come to us "stealthily." That was a visit by the "accuser of the brethren," who had a message for Job: "You are suffering because of your sin." In truth Job was suffering because "there is none like him on the earth, a blameless and upright man, who fears God and turns away from evil" (Job 1:8). Good people do suffer for the sake of righteousness.

Christians all over the world are having demonic visitations at night. They are suddenly aroused from deep sleep by an overwhelming sense of fear that makes their hair stand up. Some report a pressure on their chest, and when they try to respond they seemingly can't, as though something were grabbing their throats. At such times the presence of evil is all we sense, but God is also present. If we call upon the name of the

Lord we will be saved. For those who think, *But fear was controlling my life, and an evil force was preventing me from saying anything!* Paul answers, "The weapons of our warfare are not of the flesh but have divine power to destroy strongholds" (2 Corinthians 10:4). This is not a physical battle that requires a physical response. God knows the thoughts and intentions of your heart, so you can always turn to Him inwardly. The moment you do, you will be free to call upon the Lord. Just say "Jesus," and the attack will stop. If you submit to God first, you will be able to resist the devil and he will flee from you (James 4:7).

When I first went public with my ministry I would be visited by an evil spirit at 3 a.m. the night before every conference, and it continued for four years. How much do you think the omnipresence of God means to me? "We know that everyone who has been born of God does not keep on sinning, but he who was born of God protects him, and the evil one does not touch him. We know that we are from God, and the whole world lies in the power of the evil one" (1 John 5:18–19). It is no wonder that anxiety disorders are the number one mental health problem of the world. Fear was the first emotion that Adam acknowledged after the fall, which arose from a state of disconnection.

I'm writing this book in real time: it's like a diary of my last journey together with Joanne. As I was typing the last few paragraphs I received a call from a nurse who cares for Joanne. She said, "Your wife asked me to call you. She is afraid that she is all alone. I'm handing the phone to Joanne now." If I needed some affirmation about what I was writing, I just got it. I assured Joanne that I would be back that evening, and she said, "Oh, okay." I had been with Joanne for two hours in the morning. I had given her a shower, dried her hair, and put three types of lotion on her body. There was a general lotion for most of her body, a special lotion to ease the itching that comes from sleeping on her back, and another special lotion for her calloused feet. Huge callouses had built up on her heels just from lying in bed on her back all the time. We now put a pillow under her calves to better distribute her weight.

Why was she afraid of being alone when the nurse was standing right beside her? There are occasions when the presence of any human or even a pet makes us feel safer, and not alone. The presence of a shady person or wild animal will have the opposite effect. There are other occasions when only the presence of the right person or people can assuage our fears. Think of a frightened child on a playground, at a daycare center, or at school that can't be consoled until a parent shows up. In some cases the right parent needs to show up, which is most often the mother. Have you ever been cared for by someone who is doing it simply to make a living? The caring stops when the shift ends. Have you ever been cared for by a person who loves you voluntarily at their own expense? There is no fear when love shows up.

That phone call had an immediate impact on me. Joanne's need for my presence has kept me off the road with only rare exceptions for the last three years. During that time I have written the *Victory Series* and *Becoming a Disciple-Making Church*, which is something I might not have done if we were enjoying our retirement. Only recently have I started journaling my thoughts for this book, which I have been putting into words between visits when I got back home. I don't have to be home to do that. I can do that in her room – and so I will.

2

Suffering in His Presence

Endurance produces character, which contributes in some measure to the things which are to come, because it gives power to the hope which is within us. Nothing encourages a man to hope for blessing more than strength of a good character. No one who has led a good life worries about the future. Does our good really lie in hope? Yes, but not in human hopes, which often vanish and leave only embarrassment behind. Our hope is in God, and is therefore sure and immovable.

Chrysostom

Joanne and I were really looking forward to 2012. We had some short trips planned and other activities that we could do together. The big event was in June, when our ministry was having an international staff retreat in Bristol, England. I had run my leg of the race and I was handing off the baton to Steve Goss, our new International Director. Joanne and I had planned the trip of a lifetime. We booked a Tauck tour of Ireland, after which I would do a couple of conferences in England, then attend our international meeting. We were going to return to the States on the *Queen Mary II*.

Joanne's health began to decline right after the first of the year. In March she called off the trip, but I held on until May. Fortunately we had bought trip insurance, but it was a very disappointing time for both of us. For the next two years we searched for answers. She was poked and prodded, but there was no definitive diagnosis. She was like the "woman who had had a discharge of blood for twelve years, and who had suffered much under many physicians, and had spent all that she had, and was no better but grew worse" (Mark 5:25–26). When doctors can't find any physical cause they often assume their client is a "head" case. No psychiatric medicine, however, offered any relief. I could recognize a mild depression, but I knew it was secondary.

November 2013 was the defining moment for me. I was sitting in front of my computer and I heard from God that Joanne was not going to get well. There was no audible voice. It was an impression on my mind that came with its own authority. Frustration turned to tears, and everything changed after that. I stopped searching for answers and focused all my attention on easing her discomfort. Joanne's father had passed away with dementia, and we were not going to go down the same path that he did. While her mind was still capable of making most decisions we put all our property in my name, redid our will, and reworked our living wills.

It is a year later now, and I'm sitting in her room listening to her labored breathing. The skilled nursing facility is the best around and they have done what they can to make the environment as pleasant as possible, but death is all around us. This is the final stop for most of the residents. Some stare into space, while others struggle with aches and pains. I pay extra for a single occupancy room, and have done what I can to decorate the place. Amongst the moans and groans there is an occasional cry: "Help me. Help me." A nurse or resident assistant responds to the call, but often finds nothing physically wrong. There is an eternity of difference between Jesus saying on the cross, "I'm thirsty," which is a physical and temporal need, and "My God, my God," which is a spiritual need and an eternal cry for help. Nobody likes to suffer alone. Sadly, many do in such places.

Mature believers know that suffering is part of our sanctification. Paul says, "We rejoice in our sufferings, knowing that suffering produces endurance, and endurance produces character, and character produces hope, and hope does not put us to shame, because God's love has been poured into our hearts through the Holy Spirit who has been given to us" (Romans 5:3–5). I don't believe we have to look for opportunities to suffer in order to be like Jesus. God says He'll arrange it for us: "I form light and create darkness, I make well-being and create calamity, I am the Lord, who does all these things" (Isaiah 45:7). If He is the One who forms it, then we know He is present – even in darkness. Isaiah 50:10–11 instructs us how to navigate through the darkness:

Who among you fears the Lord and obeys the voice of his servant? Let him who walks in darkness and has no light trust in the name of the Lord and rely on his God. Behold, all you who kindle a fire, who equip yourselves with burning torches! Walk by the light of your fire, and be the torches that you have kindled! This you have from my hand: you shall lie down in torment.

Isaiah is not talking about the darkness of sin. The instruction is for those who trust in God and rely on Him. It is the darkness of uncertainty. Where there is light the path ahead is clear, but in the darkness we can easily lose our bearings. We feel lost and alone in uncharted waters. A blanket of heaviness settles in like a dark cloud. The uncertainties of tomorrow are smothering the assurances of yesterday. What should we do when God has suspended His conscious blessings? Twice before Joanne and I experienced God's ministry of darkness, and both were life-changing events.

When I was a pastor Joanne developed cataracts (as had her mother at forty years of age). In those days they would not do lens implants unless you were at least sixty years old. So both of Joanne's eyes slowly clouded over, and they removed the lens. She first had to wear those hideously thick glasses, until she could be fitted with contacts. Losing your eyesight can be traumatic in and of itself, but coupling that experience with being a pastor's wife was too much for Joanne. I knew I needed to get her out of that role, but we were in the middle of a very exciting building program. So I released her from any church obligations and promised her that I would find another way to serve God. That was my motivation to finish my first doctoral degree. I had no idea at the time what God would do with that. I was just trying to be better prepared for whatever God had in store for us.

We finished the building program and moved onto new land and into new facilities. Three months later I resigned and took a year off for study. In one year I completed forty-three semester units (seventeen of those units were Hebrew and Greek), took my comprehensive exams, did my research, and wrote my dissertation. It was a year without income, and I wanted to accomplish as much as I could. Joanne was all for it. A friend in the doctoral program promised a $20,000 interest-free loan in two installments. The plan was to finish two degrees, and then sell my home, which had enough equity to pay off the loan. I was confident that God had a place for me in His kingdom. The first six months were going as planned. Then God turned out the light.

Two weeks before my final exam I found out that the second $10,000 installment was not going to be available. The exams were only given three times a year, and only three of twenty candidates had passed the last time. I couldn't start my research unless I passed the comprehensives. I had felt sure of God's leading when I resigned from the church, but now I wondered, *Did I miss something or do something wrong?* Heaven was silent!

Our natural instinct when engulfed by darkness is to stop, sit down, drop out, or quit. God says, "Keep on walking in the light of previous revelation. If it was true last summer, it is still true. Never doubt in darkness what God has shown you in the light." But there is another, more sinister, natural response and that is to create our own light. If we don't see it God's way, we are tempted to do it *our* way. Isaiah said, "walk by the light of your own fire" and "you shall lie down in torment." The temptation to create my own light during that time was intense. I did look into two prospects, but I knew they weren't for me, and I couldn't accept them. I tried selling the house, but interest rates were near 20 percent in 1981, and there were no buyers.

It was like God had dropped us into a funnel, and when I thought it was really dark we hit the narrow part. The cupboards were literally bare. I had always thought I was a hard-working person you could count on, but now I couldn't even feed my family. It was the eleventh hour and fifty-ninth minute when God dropped us out of the funnel, and the light came back on.

We went to bed in darkness on a Thursday evening, and woke up in the middle of the night with an incredible awareness of His presence. There were no audible voices or visions, but the impressions upon my mind were crystal clear. *Do you walk by faith or do you walk by sight? Can you trust Me now? Do you love Me, or do you love My blessings? Can you worship Me now, when all the circumstances are unfavorable?* I found myself saying with a level of confidence that can't be explained apart from the presence of "the founder and perfecter of our faith" (Hebrews 12:2): *I believe You. I choose to live by faith. I love and worship You just because of who You are.* Joanne was aware that something special was going on as well. Even though our circumstances hadn't changed a bit, we both knew it was over, and indeed it was.

Such precious moments can't be planned or predicted. They're not repeatable. What we have intellectually learned from the Bible becomes incarnate. The Bible tells us what to believe, but we only really learn to trust when we are put in a position where we have to. It feels like God is dragging you through a knot hole, and just before you rip in half, you suddenly spring free on the other side, but you will never go back to the same shape you were before.

The very next day everything changed. On Friday morning I received a call from Dr. Glenn O'Neal, the Dean of Talbot School of Theology. He asked me if I had taken a position yet, and when I said no, he asked me to come by the school that afternoon. I did, and he offered me a position that I kept for the next ten years. Being a seminary professor had never previously entered my mind.

That same Friday evening a single man from the church I had been pastoring knocked on our door at 10 p.m. I said, "Chuck, what are you doing here?"

He said, "I don't know."

I said, "Come on in; we'll figure out something." During our conversation I facetiously asked, "Do you want to buy a house?"

"Maybe I do," he said. He stopped by the next Monday with his parents, and we closed the deal. Now I had the money to pay off the loan, and I knew where we were moving to. What helped us during that time was a prior commitment that we had made, and that was to never make a major decision when we are down. Impulsive decisions during a crisis can ruin one's future.

Others far greater than me have also experienced God's ministry of darkness. God had called Abraham out of Ur into the Promised Land. God made a covenant with Abraham promising that his descendants would be more numerous than the grains of sand or the stars of the sky. Abraham lived his life in the light of that promise, and then God turned out the light. So many months and years went by that Abraham's wife, Sarah, could no longer bear a child by natural means. God's guidance had been clear, but Abraham got tired of waiting and made the fatal choice of assisting God in the fulfillment of His promise. Abraham created his own light, and Sarah supplied the match by offering her handmaiden to Abraham. Because of that union the whole world lies down in torment. Jews and Arabs have struggled to live peacefully together to this day.

God superintended Moses' birth and arranged for him to be raised in the home of Pharaoh. He rose to a prominent position in Pharaoh's court. Then God put into Moses' heart a burden to set his fellow Israelites free. Impulsively, Moses killed an oppressive slave master, and God turned out the light. Abandoned to the back side of the desert, Moses spent forty years tending his father-in-law's sheep. Then one day God put the light back on. Moses turned aside to see a burning bush that wasn't being consumed. It continued to burn because God was in the bush. Moses got the message. We will burn out in a hurry if we try to serve God in our own strength and resources. If we want to be on fire for God, we had better do it by the power of His presence.

I don't think there are very many Christians mature enough to wait forty years for God to turn the light back on. God knows how big a knot hole He can pull us through. When we are stretched to our limit He pulls us through to the other side.

Our second major encounter was even more testing. Joanne's eye doctor suggested that they do a lens implant. The insurance company balked at first, saying that such a surgery was cosmetic, but they finally came around. I was excited, but Joanne was less than enthralled with the idea. I have recently had cataract surgery and I can tell you that it is discomforting to have someone cut into your eye while you are awake.

It was a day surgery, and I was in the waiting room. It seemed to be taking longer than we had been told. Finally a nurse came out and asked for my assistance. Joanne was emotionally disturbed after surgery, and they wanted my help to get her dressed and out of there. They needed the bed. They should have kept her overnight and waited for her to stabilize before sending her home. I am a great fan of the medical profession, and would have been a doctor if God hadn't called me to this present ministry, but insurance and politics don't make for good medicine.

I didn't understand at the time what Joanne was struggling with. It turns out that neither did anyone else. We were in the funnel again, going from doctor to doctor. She was hospitalized five times. If you are a forty-five-year-old female and there is no identifiable cause for your illness, you are assumed to be either a head or a hormone case. Psychiatric medications again had no impact on her condition. Our insurance ran out and we had to sell our house a second time in order to pay the medical bills. At first I thought, or was hoping, that an answer would be soon coming, but weeks turned into months.

At the time I was the chairman of the Practical Theology Department at Talbot School of Theology. I was caught in a role conflict. Was I her pastor, or counselor, or therapist, or discipler, or husband? I came to the conclusion that I could only be her husband. Somebody else would have to "fix" her. My role was to hold on to her every day and say, "This too will pass." Isaiah 21:11–12 was meaningful to me: "One is calling to me from Seir, 'Watchman, what time of the night? Watchman, what time of the night?' The watchman says: 'Morning comes, and also the night.'" No matter how dark the night, *morning comes*. If I didn't believe that I wouldn't be in ministry today.

In all honesty I felt like a modern-day Job. I even had three of his friends show up to help me out! It really stings to be accused of being the reason your spouse is sick. Most of my friends and colleagues, however, did their best to stand by us. The right help came from an older undergraduate Bible professor named Nick Kurtanick. He would wander into my office once or twice a week and ask, "Is there any change?" When I said no, he said, "Let's pray." Words are inadequate to tell you what that meant to me. Nick, himself, had been there before. He was weeks away from death fifteen years earlier, when God healed him. He knew that we are supposed to weep with those who weep, not instruct those who weep, because what we really need is the presence of God and friends. Good friends just show up. Words cannot replace presence, and the right presence doesn't need words. "A man of many companions may come to ruin, but there is a friend who sticks closer than a brother" (Proverbs 18:24).

The man who taught Pastoral Counseling in our department resigned that year. The Dean didn't want to hire any new faculty, and asked if I would teach the class. My expertise was evangelism, discipleship, leadership, management, Christian education, ethics, etc. This was a professional move that I would not have naturally made, but it turned out to be one of the biggest turning points in my life. It was also paradoxical. I was "mister fix-it" to my kids, the "go-to guy" if you wanted a problem solved, but now I had a wife that I couldn't fix. Nothing changed, no matter what I did or how I prayed. I had learned a valuable lesson of trusting God during hard times the first time around. I never made one move to create my own light, and I never once entertained any negative thoughts toward God. I kept on living in the light of previous revelation, and chose not to doubt God in the darkness, but it was still a painful and lonely time.

My ministry, however, was taking off. I was seeing God set people free, but my family was going down. My daughter Heidi wasn't sure if she could handle the death of her mother, so she had a tendency to stay away. My son Karl was very close to his mother, and it probably hit him the hardest. Joanne couldn't function as a wife or mother during that time. So I became the chief cook and bottle washer. We had moved into a modest rental that functioned as a duplex. The owners lived in part of the house. God stripped us down to nothing. All we had was God and each other. When God is all you have, you start to believe that God is all you need. After fifteen long months, morning came.

Biola University was having a day of prayer that included Talbot School of Theology. I had nothing to do with the programming other than to emphasize prayer in my classes. I was delayed on campus with a student who needed special help. I called the kids and said I wouldn't be home for dinner. The undergraduate students were having a communion service at 7 p.m. I went to the gym and sat on the floor with them. It may have been one of the loneliest times of my life. Then came Jesus. I don't remember a single word spoken at the service. I don't even remember taking communion, but I had communion with God. I was no longer alone.

There were no voices or visions, but I clearly heard from God. *Neil, there is a price to pay for freedom. Are you willing to pay the price?* We have all suffered because of personal sin and bonehead decisions, so we can't help but wonder what we have done wrong during such times of testing. *Lord, if that is the reason, I'm willing, but if my family is suffering because of my failure, please tell me.* When I left the gym that night I knew it was over, even though our circumstances hadn't changed. Within a week Joanne woke up one morning and said, "I slept last night." It was over. She never looked back.

During those dark times we can't help but wonder, *Why, God; why?* I firmly believe that He has no obligation to answer that question. *I'm God, and I can do what I want with your life, and if you don't give Me that right then I'm not your God.* Job's friends were wrong in their counsel. Job wasn't suffering because of his sin. People do suffer for the sake of righteousness. Job was wrong in defending himself, and he realized it when God asked him a hundred questions, beginning with "Where were you when I laid the foundations of the earth?" (Job 38:4f). You will know why, when morning comes.

I thought I was a caring person before that time, but not to the extent that I am now. "What is desired in a man is steadfast love (or kindness)" (Proverbs 19:22). Ask any wife which she would prefer in her husband – strong masculinity or kindness – and she will say kindness. Although that time was an important character builder, the real issue was brokenness. God brought Neil Anderson to the end of his resources so I could discover His. I had no idea how much my self-sufficient, stoic, Norwegian farming heritage was my greatest enemy to my sufficiency in Christ. I wore my self-sufficiency like a badge of honor, and would not likely have seen it as sin if God had not turned out the light – *I can tough it out. I can fix it.* Oh no we can't. Such pride will ruin us. We can't bind up the broken-hearted and set the captive free. Only God can do that, and that is why Jesus came.

That was the birth of Freedom in Christ Ministries. Every book that I have written, and every audio and visual recording I've made, was after that. I wasn't any smarter; I was just more dependent. Jesus said, "If anyone would come after me, let him deny himself and take up his cross and follow me. For whoever would save his life will lose it, but whoever loses his life for my sake will find it" (Matthew 16:24–25). What you are denying is self-rule. Jesus has to be more than your Savior if you want to experience His presence. He has to be Lord.

I don't know of any painless way to die to self, but it is the means by which we manifest His presence.

> *But we have this treasure in jars of clay, to show that the surpassing power belongs to God and not to us. We are afflicted in every way, but not crushed; perplexed, but not driven to despair; persecuted, but not forsaken; struck down, but not destroyed; always carrying in the body the death of Jesus, so that the life of Jesus may also be manifested in our bodies. For we who live are always being given over to death for Jesus' sake, so that the life of Jesus also may be manifested in our mortal flesh.* (2 Corinthians 4:7–11)

Don't feel sorry for me. It was the greatest thing that ever happened to me. What appears to be sacrificial is actually a magnificent defeat. You sacrifice the pleasure of things to gain the pleasures of life. You sacrifice the temporal to gain the eternal. The real tragedy is to seek happiness as a mortal, instead of being blessed as a child of God. What would you exchange for love, joy, peace, patience, kindness, goodness, faithfulness, gentleness, and self-control? Every child of God can have that. It comes from living in His presence. All we have to do is be filled with the Spirit, and abide in Christ.

We're in the funnel again, but this time it's different. The hard part is watching Joanne suffer. I just received a call from a resident assistant. She handed the phone to Joanne. "I can't sit up in bed," she said.

"Joanne," I replied, "you need to ask the nurse to help you with that."

She said to the assistant, "I'm supposed to ask the nurse for help."

I know what will happen this time when "morning comes" for Joanne. As for myself, I'm preparing for a new kind of loneliness.

For the last three years I've become the chief cook and bottle washer again. I actually enjoy cooking, and have become fairly good at it. When Joanne went into assisted living she routinely complained about the food. Twice when a tech was present during her complaining I said in jest, "She misses my cooking. I'm a pretty good cook, aren't I, Joanne?" She said, "Yes, you are." That is high compliment from a home economist, but in reality any home cooking is better than institutional food.

When Joanne first became ill I missed going to movies, having friends over, and dining out. There is nothing wrong with seeing a movie, or dining in a nice restaurant, but it's a shallow existence if you need entertainment to fill up your life. It took some time for the full realization of that to sink in. Elizabeth Kupler Ross reported her findings that the path to death begins with denial, then anger, then bargaining, and finally acceptance or despair. I never denied Joanne's illness, but not thinking it would lead to death is a form of denial. I went through a brief period of anger, because I thought Joanne had misused her meds. Actually she had taken way too much estrogen, but that wasn't the cause of her dementia. Many people are tempted to think that it's the sick or dying person's fault that they're not having fun anymore. I have helped numerous people in the past to forgive loved ones for getting sick or for dying and leaving them alone.

I was tempted to think, *Maybe God has someone else for me when Joanne passes.* So I started looking around for who was available. Maybe that was the bargaining phase, but I got through that, and when I did I was no longer wondering where God was! I know He is present in my life by the peace I feel. Morning has already come for me, as I am discovering on a whole new level the power of His presence. It may seem to others that caring for Joanne is all give, with nothing coming back, but nothing could be further from the truth. I wouldn't exchange the peace of God that surpasses all understanding for any fleshly indulgence. It truly is more blessed to give than to receive, because in giving you are blessed.

I can't help but wonder, however, what God has in store for me and my ministry when Joanne is no longer with me. The other periods of darkness resulted in extraordinary changes in my life and ministry. I sense that will be the case this time as well. Life with God is truly an adventure. There have been no dull moments. Thank You, Jesus.

3

Coming into His Presence

The exercise of prayer should not only be free from anger, but from all mental disturbances whatever. Prayer should be uttered from a spirit like the Spirit to whom it is sent. For a defiled spirit cannot be acknowledged by a holy Spirit, nor a sad one by a joyful one, nor a fettered one by a free one... But what reason is there to go to prayer with hands indeed washed, but the spirit foul?

Tertullian

Dementia doesn't bring out the best in folks. Joanne's father became quite belligerent as his illness progressed. Several times he hit other residents when they annoyed him. My uncle was a peaceful man who attended church all his life, but even he stepped out of character in some nasty ways before he died. Joanne complains some (mostly about the food), but she hasn't shown any meanness. I believe that speaks to her character, and to prayer. She is an innocent soul and I used to jokingly say that she only sinned once – when she married me!

I believe that Satan takes advantage of vulnerable people. I made sure Joanne and I prayed when we first entered her new living space. We renounced any activities in her room that were committed in the past that were unpleasing to God, committed the room to the Lord, commanded the devil to leave in the name of Jesus, and asked the Lord to put a hedge of protection around the room. I pray that way out loud in every hotel room I stay in as well. Doing so is just being a good steward of what God has entrusted to us. I don't want any strange spirit present in a room where I sit in silence.

Joanne will also ask for prayer for specific needs almost every time I visit: "pray that I will sleep tonight," "pray that I won't choke on my food," "pray that I won't fall or slip." Most requests are fear related, and she will occasionally say a short prayer herself. Prayer is making a conscious effort to come into God's presence. I had a blessed encounter with God many years ago that taught me how we should come into His presence.

The discipline of prayer was the most frustrating part of my early Christian experience. In seminary I read about great saints who would spend two, three, or four hours a day in prayer – sometimes all night. I had trouble spending five minutes in prayer! I would work through my prayer list for two or three minutes, glance at my watch, and then try to figure out what I was going to say for the next two minutes. I thought prayer was supposed to be a dialogue with God, but most of the time it seemed like I was talking to the wall. Why wasn't I hearing from God, and why was prayer such a mental battle? I could identify with what A. B. Simpson wrote in a little booklet entitled *Power of Stillness*:[1]

A score of years ago, a friend placed in my hand a little book which became one of the turning points of my life. It was entitled, True Peace. *It was an old medieval message, and it had but one thought, and it was this – that God was waiting in the depths of my being to talk to me if I would only get still enough to hear His voice. I thought this would be a very easy matter, and so I began to get still. But I had no sooner commenced than a perfect pandemonium of voices reached my ears,*

1   A. B. Simpson, *The Power of Stillness*, Alliance Weekly, April 16, 1916, 21.

a thousand clamoring notes from without and within, until I could hear nothing but their noise and din.

Some of them were my own voice; some of them were my own questions, some of them were my own cares, some of them were my very prayers. Others were the suggestions of the tempter and the voices of the world's turmoil. Never before did there seem so many things to be done, to be said, to be thought; and in every direction I was pushed and pulled, and greeted with noisy acclamations and unspeakable unrest. It seemed necessary for me to listen to some of them, and to answer some of them; but God said, "Be still, and know that I am God."

Then came the conflict of thoughts for tomorrow, and its duties and cares, but God said, "Be still." And as I listened, and slowly learned to obey, and shut my ears to every sound, I found after a while that when the other voices ceased, or I ceased to hear them, there was a still, small voice in the depths of my being that began to speak with an inexpressible tenderness, power, and comfort.

My prayer life changed forever one evening when I was teaching a series of lessons on prayer to a group of college students. I was basing my messages on a hundred-year-old book about prayer. The last chapter was entitled "How to Pray in the Spirit." I read the first half of the book and thought it was theologically sound. So I advertised the titles of each chapter in the book to be the subjects of my lessons that summer – not too creative, but typical of young pastors whose reservoir of wisdom is quite shallow. It takes years to internalize the whole gospel, so we teach the notes of dead saints until the message is our own. I didn't even read the last chapter of the book until the night before I was going to tell the college students how they were supposed to pray by the Spirit.

After reading that last chapter, I didn't have the foggiest idea how to pray by the Spirit (no reflection on the author of the book)! I was hours away from giving a message I had not incorporated into my own life. I felt spiritually bankrupt. I uttered a little prayer: *Need a little help down here, Lord!* If you have never been in such a spiritual state, then let me say that those times have the potential of being great moments with God.

I had all but given up trying to prepare a talk on how to pray by the Spirit and was looking around for a movie I could show. Fortunately I couldn't take the easy way out, since there were very few 16 mm movies lying around. When I was about ready to give up, then came Jesus! It was approaching midnight when the Lord began to direct my thoughts. My journey through the Bible that evening turned out to be one of the most impactful experiences of my life. I began to reason, *If I'm going to pray in the Spirit, then I must be filled with the Spirit.* So I turned in my Bible to Ephesians 5:18–20 (emphasis below is mine):

> *And do not get drunk with wine, for that is debauchery, but be filled with the Spirit, addressing one another in psalms and hymns and spiritual songs, singing and making melody to the Lord with your heart,* giving thanks always *and for everything to God the Father in the name of our Lord Jesus Christ.*

Then I turned to the parallel passage in Colossians 3:15–17:

> *And let the peace of Christ rule in your hearts, to which indeed you were called in one body. And* be thankful. *Let the word of Christ dwell in you richly, teaching and admonishing one another in all wisdom, singing psalms and hymns and spiritual songs,* with thankfulness *in your hearts to God. And whatever you do, in word or deed, do everything in the name of the Lord Jesus,* giving thanks *to God the Father through him.*

I had learned in seminary that being "filled with the Spirit" and "letting the word of Christ richly dwell" within us had the same results, but I hadn't previously observed that both were accompanied with thankfulness. I turned the page in my Bible to Colossians 4:2: "Continue steadfastly in prayer, *being watchful in it with thanksgiving*." Then I recalled Philippians 4:6: "do not be anxious about anything, but in everything by prayer and supplication *with thanksgiving*…" This discovery was fascinating as I recalled 1 Thessalonians 5:17–18: "pray without ceasing, *give thanks* in all circumstances; for this is the will of God in Christ Jesus for you." Prayer and thanksgiving seemed to be inseparable. Like a little child finding another package under the Christmas tree – and another, and another – I started looking for Paul's own personal experiences in his epistles, and this is what I found:

I do not cease to give thanks for you, remembering you in my prayers… (Ephesians 1:16)

I thank my God in all my remembrance of you, always in every prayer of mine… (Philippians 1:3–4)

We always thank God, the Father of our Lord Jesus Christ, when we pray for you... (Colossians 1:3)

We give thanks to God always for all of you, constantly mentioning you in our prayers... (1 Thessalonians 1:2)

First of all, then, I urge that supplications, prayers, intercessions, and thanksgivings be made for all people... (1 Timothy 2:1)

I thank God whom I serve, as did my ancestors, with a clear conscience, as I remember you constantly in my prayers night and day. (2 Timothy 1:3)

I thank my God always when I remember you in my prayers... (Philemon 1:4)

It was exciting to discover how important our attitude is when it comes to approaching God, but it didn't answer my bigger question: how does one pray by the Spirit? With the connection between prayer and thanksgiving established in my mind, the Lord reminded me of Psalm 95:

Oh come, let us sing to the Lord; let us make a joyful noise to the rock of our salvation! Let us come into his presence with thanksgiving; let us make a joyful noise to him with songs of praise! For the

Lord is a great God, and a great King above all gods. In his hand are the depths of the earth; the heights of the mountains are his also. The sea is his, for he made it, and his hands formed the dry land. Oh come, let us worship and bow down; let us kneel before the Lord, our Maker! For he is our God, and we are the people of his pasture, and the sheep of his hand. Today, if you hear his voice... (verses 1–7)

We should come into His presence with thanksgiving, because He is a great God and He has done great things for us. We all deserve eternal damnation, but God has forgiven us and given us eternal life. That alone should cause us to be grateful every moment of the day. However, it was the last few words in the above passage – "Today, if you hear his voice" – that really caught my attention. I remember thinking, *Today, I would love to hear Your voice!* Maybe I wasn't hearing His voice because I wasn't coming before His presence with thanksgiving. Then again, maybe I wasn't hearing His voice because I wasn't really listening.

Many people in the Old Testament discovered the hard way that complaining does not bring God's blessings. In Psalm 95:7, the word "hear" is the Hebrew word *shema*, which means "to hear as to obey." Verse 8 then reads, "Do not harden your hearts." Why would that admonishment follow? I turned to Hebrews 4:7, which quotes Psalm 95, and read again, "Today if you hear his voice, do not harden your hearts." Hebrews chapter four instructs us concerning the "Sabbath rest" that remains. It is an exhortation to cease trusting in our own works and begin trusting in God's works. The Psalmist wrote, "Seek the Lord and his strength; seek his presence continually."

Resting in the finished work of Christ did not typify my prayer life. Praying "in the name of Jesus" was just a phrase I tagged on to the end of my self-originated prayers. I confessed to God that my prayer time was mostly a work of the flesh, and that I didn't always come before Him with an attitude of praise and thanksgiving.

The Lord had a lot more for me that night. I turned to Romans 8:26–27:

> *Likewise the Spirit helps us in our weakness. For we do not know what to pray for as we ought, but the Spirit himself intercedes for us with groanings too deep for words. And he who searches hearts knows what is the mind of the Spirit, because the Spirit intercedes for the saints according to the will of God.*

Humanly speaking, we really don't know how to pray or what to pray for, but the Holy Spirit does – and He will help us in our weakness. *Sunantilambano* ("help") is a fascinating Greek word. It has two prefixes in front of a word that is often translated as "take." The Holy Spirit comes alongside us, bears us up, and takes us over to the other side (spiritually). The Holy Spirit connects us with God. He intercedes for us on our behalf. The prayer that the Holy Spirit prompts us to pray is the prayer that God the Father will always answer.

How does the Holy Spirit help us in our weakness? I wasn't sure, but I tried something that evening. I prayed, *Okay, Lord – I'm setting aside my list, and I'm going to assume that whatever comes to my mind during this time of prayer is from You or is allowed by You for a reason. I'm going to let You lead my time of prayer.* Whatever came to my mind that evening was what I prayed about. If it was a tempting thought, I talked to God about that area of weakness. If the busyness of the day clamored for my attention, I discussed my plans with God. I actively dealt with whatever came to my mind. I spent an hour in prayer for the first time in my life.

I wasn't passively letting thoughts control me. I put up the shield of faith, which stands against Satan's flaming arrows, and I was actively "[taking] every thought captive to obey Christ" (2 Corinthians 10:5).

If we don't assume responsibility for our thoughts, we may end up paying attention to a deceiving spirit, as Paul warned us: "Now the Spirit expressly says that in later times some will depart from the faith by devoting themselves to deceitful spirits and teachings of demons" (1 Timothy 4:1). Paul also wrote, "But I am afraid that as the serpent deceived Eve by his cunning, your thoughts will be led astray from a sincere and pure devotion to Christ" (2 Corinthians 11:3).

If my thoughts weren't true according to Scripture as I knew it or if they were evil (blasphemous, deceiving, accusing, or tempting), then I didn't believe them. I brought those thoughts to the Lord and exposed them to the light of His Word. In one sense, it doesn't make any difference whether our thoughts come from an external source, or from our memories, or from a deceiving spirit: we are responsible for taking every thought captive to the obedience of Christ. That meant, if my thoughts were coming from Satan, God was allowing it. In my experience, this typically identifies an area of weakness or sin that I have not previously been honest with God about. In fact, God may allow us to get buffeted around by Satan until we bring our struggles before Him, the only One who can resolve them. Psalm 90 is a prayer of Moses, and he wrote in verse 8, "You have set our iniquities before you, our secret sins in the light of your presence."

I was hearing from God, but not in the way I thought I would. I didn't want to talk to God about most of the things that came to my mind that evening, which is why we are warned not to harden our hearts. If we don't harden our hearts we will discover how personal and how present our God really is. In the past, I would try to shove evil thoughts away... without much success. But when I began to bring them to the light, I was amazed at how liberating that was. All the issues I had been trying to ignore during prayer were issues God wanted me to deal with. He wanted to make me aware of matters that were affecting our relationship. Now, when I have tempting or accusing thoughts, I'm honest with God and don't try to hide my human frailties.

When a thought that's hard to face comes into our mind, we will be tempted to change the subject and go back to our old prayer list. Why do you think God is allowing us to struggle with those thoughts? There may be many personal issues that we feel uncomfortable sharing with God, but that is part of the deception. God already knows our thoughts:

For the Word of God is living and active, sharper than any two-edged sword, piercing to the division of soul and of spirit, of joints and of marrow, and

*discerning the thoughts and intentions of the heart.
And no creature is hidden from his sight, but all
are naked and exposed to the eyes of him to whom
we must give account. (Hebrews 4:12–13)*

We are already forgiven, so why not be honest with
Him? If we let God prioritize our prayer list, He
will begin with the personal issues that affect our
relationship with Him.

Suppose you are a parent who has a rebellious
child and there are several unresolved issues that are
keeping you from having an intimate relationship.
Immature children come to a parent with a list of
requests, most of which are geared to the satisfaction
of their own desires – *I want this, I want that, and
can I go there*? As you listen to their petitions, what
is on your mind as a loving parent? Satisfying their
desires and giving them what they request will spoil
the child. It is not good for their maturation, and it
will not improve your relationship with the child. You
want to look after their needs, and you know better
than trying to satisfy their fleshly desires. As a mature
adult, you want to share with the child what is best for
them, but they don't want to listen to you. So what do
you do? What does God do?

As children of God we are equipped with the
"mind of Christ" (1 Corinthians 2:16), and have

been given the Holy Spirit to guide us into all truth. Two members of the Trinity are actively participating with us in prayer all the time. The Holy Spirit is interceding for us and so is Jesus. "He is able to save to the uttermost those who draw near to God through him, since he always lives to make intercession for them" (Hebrews 7:25). The only impediment to the process of real prayer is ourselves.

After explaining what it means to pray by the Spirit in seminary classes, I directed the students to take a walk around the campus with God for the remainder of the class period. That would give them about forty-five minutes, which was far more time than most of them would spend in their daily devotions. I encouraged them to start by thanking God for all He had done for them. I encouraged them to deal honestly with any issues that came to their minds. If nothing came to mind, then I encouraged them to reflect upon God's goodness and thank Him for what He had done for them.

Many students returned with great stories. Some said they had accomplished more in those forty-five minutes than they ever had before in prayer. Some dealt with personal issues that they had never discussed with God previously. One Asian student said he knew for the first time that God was calling him to minister in China. Almost all found it to be a refreshing encounter with their loving heavenly Father.

As I began to put this understanding into practice myself, I found the freedom of just sitting in the presence of God. I didn't feel like I had to say anything or keep a one-sided conversation going. It was actually refreshing, and I could simply sit in silence for an hour or more. I also discovered that my prayer time didn't end when I got up to do something else. I was learning to pray without ceasing, which is essentially the same as practicing the presence of God. The omnipresent God was always with me, and I was becoming more aware of it.

Have you ever noticed that silence is awkward when you are alone with a stranger? You feel obligated to say something. So you mention the weather or the latest news and sports, but nothing personal. On the other hand, I can sit in the same room with Joanne and not feel obligated to say anything. We are comfortable in the presence of each other. How well you can handle solitude is probably the best way to determine your spiritual condition. How comfortable are you in the presence of God? Can you be still and know that He is God?

Effective communication takes place when all parties are listening. I believe that prayer is more about listening than talking. It makes me wonder whether church prayer meetings would be more effective if the first half of the allotted time was restricted to listening. If sitting silently before the Lord is awkward, then you may want to consider how intimate your relationship with God really is.

Why is it so difficult to be honest with God? He demonstrated His love for us when He sent Jesus to die in our place (Romans 5:8). His love and forgiveness are unconditional. God is our Father, and like any good parent, He doesn't appreciate grumbling, complaining children, especially since He sacrificed His only begotten Son for every one of them. He will not be interested in our prayer lists if we aren't trusting and obeying Him. He is not going to help us develop our own kingdoms when we are called to establish His kingdom!

Someone said that "prayer is not conquering God's reluctance, but laying hold of God's willingness." It is not trying to communicate our will to God, but discerning His will for our lives. Those who seek to build His kingdom and come before His presence with thanksgiving understand that "… we do not have a high priest who is unable to sympathize with our weaknesses, but one who in every respect has been tempted as we are, yet without sin. Let us then with confidence draw near to the throne of grace, that we may receive mercy and find grace to help in time of need" (Hebrews 4:15–16). "Seek the Lord and his strength; seek his presence continually" (Psalm 105:4).

In everything give thanks. The operative word is *in*. I don't thank God that my wife is slowly dying. I thank God that He is present with us. That He called us to Himself forty-six years ago. That He forgave us. That He gave us new life in Christ. That He never left us and has never forsaken us. That He has met all our needs according to His riches in glory. That He has gone before us and prepared a place for us. None of that I deserved. I am so thankful for the forty-nine years that we have had together. My heart is filled with gratitude that I can sit by my wife in His presence with a quiet mind and peaceful spirit. "Surely the righteous shall give thanks to your name; the upright shall dwell in your presence" (Psalm 140:13).

4

Ministering in His Presence

The shepherd of sheep has the flock following him wherever he leads; or if some turn aside from the direct path and leave the good pasture to graze in barren and precipitous places, it is enough for him to call more loudly, lead them back again and restore to the flock those that were separated. But if a man wanders away from the right path, the shepherd needs a lot of concentration, perseverance and patience. He cannot drag by force or constrain by fear, but must by persuasion lead him back to the true beginning from which he has fallen away. He needs, therefore, a heroic spirit, not to grow despondent or neglect the salvation of wanderers but to keep on thinking and saying, "God perhaps may give them the knowledge of the truth and they may be freed from the snare of the devil."

Chrysostom

I love my wife more now than I ever have before, but not in the way I first loved her. I was attracted to Joanne the first time I saw her. She turned me on. I liked her personality and her laugh. She was a classy lady. Attraction is a natural response when somebody else pleases you by their appearance or actions. Jesus said, "If you love those who love you, what benefit is that to you? For even sinners love those who love them" (Luke 6:32). Now Joanne can't do anything for me. Victims of dementia don't consider other people more important than themselves (Philippians 2:3). The only needs they are aware of are their own, and Joanne's needs dominate our time together: "I need a Kleenex." "Get me some water." "I need to go to the bathroom." Occasionally she says "thank you." When I need to leave I often hear, "Please don't leave." But I have to, and I have learned not to feel guilty when I do.

Think of it as parental love for a newborn baby. I will never forget when our daughter Heidi was born. I wanted to hold her, kiss her, provide for her, and protect her. Why? She had no personality at all. She was toothless, hairless, and helpless. She cried and complained about anything that caused her the slightest discomfort. She spit up on me when I burped her, and pooped in her pants. When I went to change the diaper, she urinated on me. She never said, "Thank you, Daddy, for changing my dirty stinking diaper." All the love was one way. Now I'm doing the same for my wife of forty-nine years, but with a lot more peace in my heart, and more time to give. From the day we first met I loved Joanne for who *she* was. Now, thanks to Jesus, I love Joanne for who I am "in Him."

Joanne can't get out of bed by herself or out of a chair, so I have to take her by both hands and pull her up. She is very feeble now as we stand face to face. Her posture makes her inches shorter. "Do you want a hug?" I ask. "All the time," she answers. She is like a little child and I find myself wanting to hold her, kiss her, provide for her, and protect her. Who wouldn't do the same if they saw a frightened little child who is afraid to be alone? Life has come full circle. She only has a short time left on this earth, and I don't want her to think for a second that she is residing in a skilled nursing facility because I no longer want her at home, or I don't care for her.

God loves us, because God is love (*agape*). When used as a noun, *agape* refers to the character of God. "Love is patient and kind; love… endures all things. Love never ends" (1 Corinthians 13:4–8). The love of God is not dependent upon the object, which is why it is unconditional. If we gave nothing back He would still love us, because it's His nature to love us. "God shows his love for us in that while we were still sinners, Christ died for us" (Romans 5:8). A husband is supposed to love his wife as Christ loved the church.

When used as a verb, *agapeo* is all give. "For God so loved the world that he gave his only Son…" (John 3:16). The sequel to that verse is 1 John 3:16–18:

> *By this we know love, that he laid down his life for us, and we ought to lay down our lives for the brothers. But if anyone has the world's goods and sees his brother in need, yet closes his heart against him, how does God's love abide in him? Little children, let us not love in word or talk but in deed and in truth.*

It is the presence of God in our lives that enables us to love others and expect nothing in return from them. On the other hand, it is one of life's great compensations that we cannot truly help another without helping ourselves in the process.

Christians are God's children, but every struggling believer that I have had the privilege to work with has had one thing in common. None of them knew who they were in Christ, nor did they understand what it meant to be a child of God. Those who have not resolved their personal and spiritual conflicts have little awareness of God's presence. If "the Spirit himself bears witness with our spirit that we are children of God" (Romans 8:16), why aren't many believers sensing that? Tragically, what they are sensing is a lot of mental and emotional conflict. Sitting alone in silence is intolerable for those who have no mental peace. They have to constantly be doing something to keep their minds occupied, or they drown out their thoughts with alcohol or drugs. Nobody wants to share what is going on in their mind with others, so they suffer alone. Many think they are the only ones who struggle with their thoughts.

The precipitating cause is usually fractured relationships – first with God and then with each other. We have all been wounded at some time in our lives by others. Wounds that are not transformed are transferred to others. It took me years to learn that people are not in bondage to past traumas; they are in bondage to the lies they believed because of the trauma. Adding insult to injury, the devil accuses, tempts, and deceives the whole world (Revelation 12:9). "The Spirit expressly says that in later times some will depart from the faith by devoting themselves to deceitful spirits and teachings of demons" (1 Timothy 4:1). That is presently happening all over the world.

Where is the presence of God?

In my early years of ministry I believed God was the answer, and truth would set people free, but I saw very little evidence of God's presence. The Bible tells us that God is present, but it also tells us that "the whole world lies in the power of the evil one" (1 John 5:19). I had introduced a lot of people to Christ, and I saw some change, but most seemed to struggle with many of the same old issues. When I was called to teach at Talbot School of Theology, I went there with a burden: How is Christ the answer and how does truth set one free? Little did I know that God was about to lead me through some major paradigm shifts.

In my first pastoral ministry I started a school of evangelism. I saw hundreds come to Christ, and that confirmed to me that the field really was white unto harvest. So, when I first taught evangelism at Talbot School of Theology, I thought I had a pretty good handle on what constituted the gospel; but I didn't. Of course I believed in the resurrection, but all my emphasis was on the cross. We had all sinned and fallen short of the glory of God, and needed to be forgiven. Sin had separated us from God. So Jesus had voluntarily marched to the cross and died for our sins. A great chasm existed between God and humanity, and the cross bridged that gap.

What I didn't fully understand at the time was that what Adam and Eve lost in the fall was *life*, and that is what Jesus came to give us (John 10:10). One day the scales fell from my eyes, and I realized that I was spiritually alive in Christ. My soul was in union with God. Oh, what a glorious day that was! I may have known that theologically, but now I knew that God was my Father and I was His child. "But to all who did receive him, who believed in his name, he gave the right to become children of God, who were born, not of blood nor of the will of the flesh nor of the will of man, but of God" (John 1:12–13).

In evangelism I had used the questions of the late pastor and televangelist James Kennedy: "If you died tonight, do you know where you would spend eternity?" "What would you say if you appeared before God and were asked, 'What right do you have to be here?'?" I knew it was only by the grace of God that I had any right to be in His presence. The first question had the right intent, and often opened the door for a gospel presentation. However, where we spend eternity is not the essential issue, because eternal life is not something we get when we die. I have no idea where heaven is, but I do know that it is a state of being fully in God's presence. When we die physically, we will be absent from the body and present with the

Lord (2 Corinthians 5:8). The assurance of our eternal state is based on what we have now, "which is Christ in you, the hope of glory" (Colossians 1:27). "And this is the testimony, that God gave us eternal life, and this life is in his Son. Whoever has the Son has life; whoever does not have the Son of God does not have life" (1 John 5:11–12). The presence of God is now in those who are born again in a new way that He wasn't before. So why doesn't every believer know that?

God said, "My people are destroyed for lack of knowledge" (Hosea 4:6), which may be one reason we don't know who we are. The truth can't set you free if you don't know it. But I think there is another reason that is more prominent. Jesus said, "The time is fulfilled, and the kingdom of God is at hand; repent and believe in the gospel" (Mark 1:15). Jesus didn't only die for our sins; He came to give us life, and He came to undo the works of the devil (1 John 3:8). Those are the three essential elements of the gospel, which is summarized in Colossians 2:13–15:

> And you, who were dead in your trespasses and the uncircumcision of your flesh, God made alive together with him, having forgiven us all our trespasses, by canceling the record of debt that stood against us with its legal demands. This he set aside, nailing it to the cross. He disarmed the rulers

and authorities and put them to open shame, by triumphing over them in him.

Christians would live differently if they knew that they were forgiven, that their souls were in union with God, and that Satan and his demons need not be feared, because they had been disarmed. However, what is missing all over the world is repentance. The moment we receive Christ, every aspect of the gospel is true, but if we want to experience our new life and freedom we have to repent. When I help believers genuinely repent and believe the gospel, their eyes are opened and they sense the presence of God bearing witness with their spirit that they are children of God. Not only do they know who they are, their minds are quiet. Most experience the peace of God in a way they have never known before. You know God is present when you see Him set captives free and heal their wounds right in front of you. If you have never seen that, let me share how that can happen, and I believe should be happening, in every church.[2]

Struggling believers usually have a distorted concept of God, they question God's love for them, and they don't have a clue who they are in Christ.

---

2   In my book, *Becoming a Disciple-Making Church* (Bethany House, 2016), I share how obstacles that impede Christians from growing can be overcome through genuine repentance and faith in God, and how they can become like Jesus.

God obviously anticipated that would be the case, which is why He inspired Paul to pray twice that our eyes would be opened to the truth:

I do not cease to give thanks for you, remembering you in my prayers, that the God of our Lord Jesus Christ, the Father of glory, may give you the Spirit of wisdom and of revelation in the knowledge of him, having the eyes of your hearts enlightened, that you may know what is the hope to which he has called you, what are the riches of his glorious inheritance in the saints. (Ephesians 1:16–18)

For this reason I bow my knees before the Father, from whom every family in heaven and on earth is named, that according to the riches of his glory he may grant you to be strengthened with power through his Spirit in your inner being, so that Christ may dwell in your hearts through faith – that you, being rooted and grounded in love, may have strength to comprehend with all the saints what is the breadth and length and height and depth, and to know the love of Christ that surpasses knowledge, that you may be filled with all the fullness of God. (Ephesians 3:14–19)

Discovering who I am in Christ was my first major paradigm shift, which I had to comprehend in order to process the next one. God was sending me all kinds of people with all kinds of problems. I would do my best to help them, but inevitably I would get stuck. James wrote, "If any of you lacks wisdom, let him ask God, who gives generously to all without reproach, and it will be given to him" (1:5). So I would tell the person, "I don't know how to help you, but I know God does. So I am going to pray, asking God for wisdom." After I had prayed out loud, I would wait upon the Lord. Sometimes I waited several minutes.

Being dependent upon God was essential, but the person I was trying to help needed to be dependent upon God as well. All temptation is an attempt by the enemy to entice us to live independently from God. James was instructing us to ask for wisdom for ourselves, not for somebody else. Every believer should ask for wisdom themselves. They are children of God, and have the same access to our heavenly Father as I do. I was asking God to tell me, so I could tell them. That would make me a medium. Paul wrote that God "desires all people to be saved and to come to the knowledge of the truth. For there is one God, and there is one mediator between God and men, the man Christ Jesus" (1 Timothy 2:4–5). With that in mind I thought, *Why don't I have them pray?* When I did, the presence of God was operative.

Suppose you have two sons, and the younger brother is always asking his older brother to petition you on his behalf: "Go ask Dad if I can go to the movies tonight." No good parent would accept a secondhand relationship with one of their children. They would likely say, "Go tell your brother to come ask me himself." I think that is what our heavenly Father is saying to all His children: *Come ask Me yourself.* "Ask, and it will be given to you; seek, and you will find; knock, and it will be opened to you. For everyone who asks receives, and the one who seeks finds, and to the one who knocks it will be opened" (Matthew 7:7–8). Nobody can do that for another person, but we can help one another.

One afternoon I wrote out several petitions that I would have inquirers pray. I sat on the idea for a while, then one afternoon I tried it. I was totally surprised at what happened. God showed them whom they needed to forgive. He brought back suppressed memories of former abuses and personal sin. He revealed their pride and rebellion. The Holy Spirit was leading them into all truth, and that truth was setting them free. In short, God was granting them repentance that removed the barriers to their intimacy with Him. Instead of feeling condemned at the end, they felt free and profoundly grateful. I couldn't help but think, *What an incredible ministry. I just helped this person become reconciled to God, who brought to light all their sins and iniquities, and they can't stop thanking me for it.* Those prayers became the "Steps to Freedom in Christ," which are being used all over the world to liberate the body of Christ.

When the opportunity arises for me to help another believer, I do so with the confidence that God is present, and that I am ministering to one of His children. I could spend the rest of my life trying to figure that person out, while God knows every minute detail about them. So doesn't it make sense that He should be included in the process? Picture a triangle with God at the top. The other two corners represent the encourager and the enquirer. Every side of the triangle represents a relationship. Now ask yourself a question. Who is responsible for what? There is a role that God and only God can play in the inquirer's life. If I usurp God's role, and try to play the role of the Holy Spirit in the other person's life, I will misdirect their battle with God unto myself.

Have you ever tried to play the role of the Holy Spirit in the life of your spouse? How did that work out for you? Have you ever tried to assume the responsibility of the person you are trying to help? If they choose not to believe, can you believe for them?

If they won't repent, can you repent for them? A lot of problems would be resolved in our churches and families if we all assumed responsibility for our own attitudes and actions. Seeking someone to do it for us won't work. The one player in the triangle that will be absolutely faithful, fully present, and responsible is God. God will faithfully execute His role, whether we do or not, but He won't repent or believe for us.

As an encourager the most important of the three relationships is the one I have with my heavenly Father. It is my first responsibility to make sure that there are no unresolved issues between me and God. A man brought his son to Jesus and said, "'I begged your disciples to cast it [a demon] out, but they could not.' Jesus answered, 'O faithless and twisted generation, how long am I to be with you and bear with you?'" (Luke 9:40–41). God cannot work through unbelieving and unrepentant encouragers.

How we are to regard inquirers, knowing what our role is and what we are trying to accomplish, is summed up in 2 Corinthians 5:16–20:

> From now on, therefore, we regard no one according to the flesh. Even though we once regarded Christ according to the flesh, we regard him thus no longer. Therefore, if anyone is in Christ, he is a new creation. The old has passed away; behold the

new has come. All this is from God, who through Christ reconciled us to himself and gave us the ministry of reconciliation; that is, in Christ God was reconciling the world to himself, not counting their trespasses against them, and entrusting to us the message of reconciliation. Therefore, we are ambassadors for Christ, God making his appeal through us. We implore you on behalf of Christ, be reconciled to God.

Paul never recognizes believers by their flesh patterns. He always recognizes believers for who they are in Christ. Christian inquirers are not alcoholics, addicts, perverts, derelicts, bums, scum, or gay. They are children of God. We don't count their trespasses against them, and there is no need to point them out, because that is God's role. He will convict the world of sin. Our role is to help them believe and repent, which removes the barriers to their intimacy with God. They experience God's presence when they pray and God shows them what they need to repent of. When God brings conviction, the power to change comes with it. If I try to correct them, they become defensive.

Struggling believers don't feel good about themselves. That could be the result of verbal abuse from others, or it could be the devil accusing them (who accuses us before God day and night [Revelation

12:10]), or they could be sensing godly conviction for their sins. Paul clarifies the difference in 2 Corinthians 7:9–10: "I rejoice, not because you were grieved, but because you were grieved into repenting. For you felt a godly grief, so that you suffered no loss through us. For godly grief produces a repentance that leads to salvation without regret, whereas worldly grief produces death." I know God is present when I see an inquirer remorseful for their sins, because that leads to repentance and the assurance of salvation. If they sense no remorse for sin, then they should question their salvation.

When they ask God what they need to repent of, God shows them, and intimate details come out in the process. God is surfacing those issues for the purpose of resolving them. If people share intimate details without resolution, they will probably regret it later. But when they do so with resolution there is no regret. There is only gratitude. Notice the difference between godly sorrow and Satan's accusations in the lives of Judas and Peter. "Satan entered into Judas" (Luke 22:3), and he betrayed Christ. He came under worldly grief and committed suicide. Peter betrayed Christ three times, came under the conviction of the Holy Spirit, and became the early spokesperson for the church.

The remaining side of the triangle is the relationship between the encourager and the inquirer. The quote by Chrysostom at the beginning of this chapter comes from his commentary on 2 Timothy 2:24–26, which explains the role of the encourager:

> *And the Lord's servant must not be quarrelsome but kind to everyone, able to teach, patiently enduring evil, correcting his opponents with gentleness. God may perhaps grant them repentance leading to a knowledge of the truth, and they may come to their senses and escape from the snare of the devil, after being captured by him to do his will.*

A servant is one who does the will of his master. We need to be dependent upon God, and not usurp His role. This kind of ministry is an encounter with God. Quarreling is a smokescreen that diverts the process away from resolution. The wise encourager keeps the process on track. The most essential character prerequisite is kindness. One act of unkindness and the process is over. The inquirer will clam up, and the session ends. They need to sense that there is not one thing they couldn't share with us, that just by sharing it wouldn't cause us to love them less; it would actually enable us to love them more.

"Able to teach" does not refer to one's ability to communicate. The focus is more on the content. We

o know the truth, because truth is what sets
e. People are in bondage to lies they believe,
and it takes patience to root out embedded lies. The
standard fifty-minute counseling session doesn't work
for this kind of ministry. We shouldn't open someone's
wounds unless we are willing to stay with the person
until they are closed.

We also have to treat people gently. We can't force
people to repent. I don't try to coerce or manipulate
anyone. It is their choice and I respect that. If they
choose to believe a lie, and fail to deal with their
issues, we have to accept it. That seldom happens, but
when it does I tell them my door is always open. They
are welcome to come back at any time. Some people
just aren't ready.

Satan will not like to lose ground, so I expect
some opposition, but we never have to lose control
of the session, because God is present. All authority
has been given to Jesus in heaven and upon this
earth. We have all the authority and power we need
because of our position in Christ. Satan likes to work
undercover, which is why the battle is in the mind. I
say to inquirers:

*Your mind is your control center; we won't lose
control in our time together if you don't lose control
of your mind. If you are having thoughts contrary*

to what we are doing, share them with me. It is just a thought and it has no power over you unless you believe it. As soon as you expose it to the light the power is broken. When we are done your mind will be quiet, but I need your cooperation. You will be asking God to reveal to your mind the problems of the past. When He does, don't harden your heart. Be as honest as you can for your sake. He loves you, and wants you free. If you get rid of the garbage the flies will leave.

This passage begins with dependence upon God, and ends with God granting repentance. The Holy Spirit was sent to lead us into all truth, and that is what enables us to escape from the snare of the devil. I always encourage the inquirer to close their eyes when we are done. Then I ask, "Is your mind quiet? Do you feel God's peace?" Ninety-five percent of the time they respond in joy. One person said, "How did you know that would happen!" There are probably several reasons why the 5 percent don't sense complete resolution, but I never put the blame on them. Usually I say, "Would you be willing to close your eyes again, and this time ask God to show you what is still keeping you from experiencing the peace and freedom He wants you to have?" Often God will take them back to defining moments in their life.

I always feel an overwhelming sense of joy and peace when I see God in action. In many cases the countenance of the person has changed so much that I suggest they go to the restroom, freshen up, and take a good look at themselves in the mirror. I feel just as blessed working with one individual as I do speaking to thousands. I'm an encourager. That is my gift. I have spoken all over the world, and I thank God for the privilege, but nothing is more satisfying than facilitating a process that sets captives free and heals the wounds of the abused.

That is why I am at peace visiting Joanne twice a day. She needs encouragement, and I am the only one who can give her that. Joanne sat in with me a couple of times with a pastor's daughter who had been ritually abused. It wasn't her father who had abused her, but he hadn't protected her and was unable to help her. Then a counselor took advantage of her sexually. She attended one of my conferences and couldn't process anything I shared. I promised to meet with her the following Monday. The following Christmas she gave us a very special gift. Hanging in my office at home is a handmade wreath, with the following inscription in the center:

A friend of mine whose grapevine died, had put it out for trash.
I said to her, I'll take that vine and make something of that.

At home the bag of dead, dry vines looked nothing but a mess.
But as I gently bent one vine, entwining 'round and 'round,

A rustic wreath began to form, potential did abound.
One vine would not go where it should, and anxious as I was,

I forced it so to change its shape, it broke — and what the cause?
If I had taken precious time to slowly change its form,

It would have made a lovely wreath, not a dead vine, broken, torn.
As I finished bending, adding blooms, applying trim,

I realized how that rustic wreath is like my life within.
You see, so many in my life have tried to make me change.

They've forced my spirit anxiously, I tried to rearrange.
But when the pain was far too great, they forced my fragile form.

I plunged far deeper in despair, my spirit broken, torn.
Then God allowed a gentle one that knew of dying vines,

To kindly, patiently allow the Lord to take His time.
And though the vine has not yet formed a decorative wreath,

I know that with God's servant's help one day when Christ I meet,
He'll see a finished circle, a perfect gift to Him.

It will be a final product, a wreath with all the trim.
So as you look upon this gift, the vine round and complete,

Remember God is using you to gently shape His wreath.

5

Resting in His Presence

Our heart is restless until it rests in God.

Augustine

Joanne and I could have been poster children for Gary Chapman's book, *The Five Love Languages.*[3] We had been happily married for thirty-five years when it was first published. After reading the book I had no doubt that my love language was service, and Joanne's was time. There couldn't have been a worse combination for us, because I was away from home a lot doing ministry around the world. When I was home I would do anything for Joanne. "Do you want the bedroom repainted? Consider it done... The toilet is blocked? I'll get the plunger. What else would you

---

3   Gary Chapman, *The Five Love Languages: How to Express Heartfelt Commitment to Your Mate* (Chicago: Northfield Publishing, 1992)

like me to do for you?" Joanne would reply: "I just want you to spend some time with me." "Certainly. What would you like to do?" *Earth to Neil!*

I still serve Joanne, but I am much more present than I was when I was establishing my career in engineering and ministry. In turn, she also has come to appreciate the way I show my love for her. I normally wake up Joanne at 6:50 for breakfast, but this morning I attended a prayer meeting, so I was late getting to the extended care center. I was very disappointed to find her still in bed at 9 a.m. Her nightgown and all the bedding were soiled. Her food was lying cold on a serving table. She should have been helped out of bed and cleaned up by 7 a.m. She doesn't know how to use the device that signals for help, so she was feebly calling for it, but nobody was responding. If you are paying $9,300 per month, you would hope for a little better care than that.

She was so relieved when I walked through the door. I took one look, walked back into the hall, and reported her condition to a tech as calmly as I could. I let God do the convicting, but I did make it clear that I would take care of her that morning. I didn't want any tension in her room. A calming presence is what she needed. I helped her to the bathroom, cleaned her up, reheated her food, sat her in a chair, and changed her bedding while she ate. It is times like these that you really need to put into practice the presence of God. A simple reprimand by the nurse on duty would be appropriate, which should be done for the purpose of ensuring better care for others and protecting the reputation of the skilled nursing facility. The last thing I want is to establish an adversarial relationship with those who are caring for Joanne.

Moses also had to deal with difficult people. He went up the mountain to receive instruction from God concerning His people. When he was delayed in coming down the people grew restless and decided to make a god for themselves in the form of a golden calf. Then God instructed Moses to go back down the mountain, because the people had corrupted themselves. So Moses picked up the two tablets that "were the work of God, and the writing was the writing of God" (Exodus 32:16). When Moses saw the rebellion he threw the tablets and broke them at the foot of the mountain. Then Moses stood at the gate and said, "Who is on the Lord's side?" (verse 26). The Levites gathered around him, and Moses ordered them to slay those who weren't. Three thousand died that day. That was not a calming presence!

Then God commanded Moses to depart from Sinai:

Moses said to the Lord, "See, you say to me, 'Bring up this people,' but you have not let me know whom you will send with me. Yet you have said, 'I know you by name, and you have also found favor in my sight.' Now therefore, if I have found favor in your sight, please show me now your ways, that I may know you in order to find favor in your sight. Consider too that this nation is your people." And he said, "My presence will go with you, and I will give you rest." (Exodus 33:12–14)

God's presence radically changed how Moses dealt with rebellious people, and he was tested three times.

When Miriam and Aaron spoke against Moses, God brought judgment upon them, but Moses interceded on their behalf (see Numbers 12:1f). When all the people of Israel grumbled against Moses, God said to Moses, "I will strike them with the pestilence and disinherit them, and I will make of you a nation greater and mightier than they" (Numbers 14:12). What leader would pass that test today? *Good for You, God; give them what they deserve, and You made a great choice in choosing me!* Moses again asked God to withhold judgment for the sake of His reputation. Finally, his leadership rebelled against him (see Numbers 16:1f), and God said He was going to bring judgment against all the congregation.

But Moses prayed, asking that the congregation be spared (verse 22). In each case judgment still came, but less severely. We live differently in the presence of God. A natural man doesn't ask God to withhold judgment when his staff, board, and congregation rebel against him, especially when he knows God wants to bring judgment. If they had never agreed with God before, they probably would on such occasions. Later in history God was looking for a man like Moses, but there was none. "I sought for a man among them who should build up the wall and stand in the breach before me for the land, that I should not destroy it, but I found none" (Ezekiel 22:30). The Temple was destroyed and the people were exiled to Babylon.

Did God give Moses rest? Obviously God's idea of rest was not an abdication of responsibility, nor a cessation of labor. For the next forty years he wandered around the wilderness with five million grumbling Jews. There was no accommodation with showers or toilets. There was only one item of food listed on the menu, and every day it was the same. That is about as restful as taking the grandchildren to Disneyland for a week, albeit less expensive. However, the quality of rest can only be assessed by how we feel at the end. "Moses was 120 years old when he died. His eye was undimmed, and his vigor unabated" (Deuteronomy 34:7). God gave him rest!

The key to biblical rest is the presence of God. Moses had already failed at serving God when he slew the Egyptian. God's people were not going to be delivered that way. "Not by might, nor by power, but by my Spirit, says the Lord of hosts" (Zechariah 4:6). Being exiled to the back side of the desert for forty years does something to a proud man. "Now the man Moses was very meek, more than all people who were on the face of the earth" (Numbers 12:3). Out of his brokenness Moses learned to do it God's way, and in His strength. Pride is what kicked Lucifer out of heaven, and pride will keep us from experiencing God's presence, because God is opposed to the proud. However, God does permit us to boast in one thing. "Let not the wise man boast in his wisdom, let not the mighty man boast in his might, let not the rich man boast in his riches, but let him who boasts boast in this, that he understands and knows me, that I am the Lord who practices steadfast love, justice, and righteousness in the earth. For in these things I delight, declares the Lord" (Jeremiah 9:23–24). The same sentiment is shared in the New Testament: "Let the one who boasts, boast in the Lord" (1 Corinthians 1:31).

Those who really know God and rely upon Him, however, are not inclined to boast. Jesus said we will know them by their fruit. "By this is my Father glorified, that you bear much fruit and so prove to be my disciples" (John 15:8). We will be like the proud Moses if we conclude that we have to bear fruit and make every effort to do so. What we have to do is abide in Christ, and rest in His finished work. Jesus said, "I am the vine; you are the branches. Whoever abides in me and I in him, he it is that bears much fruit, for apart from me you can do nothing" (John 15:5). Fruit is the evidence that we are abiding in Christ. Abiding in Christ is living God's way and in His strength.

The glory of God is a manifestation of His presence. God uniquely manifested Himself to Moses, and in the Holy of Holies. Ezekiel writes about the progressive departure of the glory of God from Judah. *Shekinah* (literally, that which dwells) is a non-biblical term that appeared in the Targums and later the Talmud to describe the presence of God. In Ezekiel the *Shekinah* glory moves back and forth from the Holy of Holies to the periphery of the city until finally the glory has departed. God didn't significantly manifest His presence again until "the Word became flesh and dwelt among us, and we have seen his glory, glory as of the only Son from the Father, full of grace and truth" (John 1:14). Jesus was the perfect manifestation of God. Jesus said, "Whoever has seen me has seen the Father" (John 14:9).

The glory of God departed again when Jesus went to be with the Father, but His glory returned at Pentecost to reside in His children: "To them God chose to make known how great among the Gentiles are the riches of the glory of this mystery, which is Christ in you, the hope of glory" (Colossians 1:27); "You are not your own, for you were bought with a price. So glorify God in your body" (1 Corinthians 6:19–20); and "do all to the glory of God" (1 Corinthians 10:31). We do that when we live by faith according to what God says is true in the power of the Holy Spirit. The fruit of the Spirit is a manifestation of God's presence in our lives. The "fruit of the Spirit is love, joy, peace, patience, kindness, goodness, faithfulness, gentleness, self-control; against such things there is no law" (Galatians 5:22–23). We can't legislate that, but nobody can keep us from being the people God created us to be, and that is God's will for our lives – to be like Jesus. Jesus said, "By this all people will know that you are my disciples, if you have love for one another" (John 13:35).

Jesus is the truth and God is love. Without the love of God we would never know the truth. Without the truth we would never know the love of God. We cannot diminish one attribute of God without distorting the others. When we disjoin love from the character of God, we diminish truth, and liberty becomes license. There will be a progressive departure of God's glory from churches and denominations that compromise God's word in the name of "love." On the other hand, God is not glorified when truth is not spoken in love. "This 'knowledge' puffs up, but love builds up" (1 Corinthians 8:1). We can know theology and be arrogant, but we can't know God and be arrogant. "The aim of our charge is love that issues from a pure heart and a good conscience and a sincere faith" (1 Timothy 1:5).

Paul strikes the balance between legalism and license in his letter to the Galatians:

> But I say, walk by the Spirit, and you will not gratify the desires of the flesh. For the desires of the flesh are against the Spirit, and the desires of the Spirit are against the flesh, for these are opposed to each other, to keep you from doing the things you want to do [license]. But if you are led by the Spirit, you are not under the law [legalism]. (5:16–18)

To live by the Spirit is neither legalism nor license. It is liberty. "Now the Lord is the Spirit, and where the Spirit of the Lord is, there is freedom" (2 Corinthians 3:17). There will be no peace for those who are stuck in the bondage of legalism or the immorality of license. Godly sorrow is the only way they will sense God's presence, which hopefully leads them to repentance (see 2 Corinthians 9:9–10). If we can't live with people, then we are not walking with God. If we can't live with ourselves, then we are not listening to God.

If you are not experiencing the presence of God and find yourself huffing and puffing your way to burnout, then listen to Jesus' words in Matthew 11:28–30: "Come to me, all who labor and are heavy laden, and I will give you rest. Take my yoke upon you, and learn from me, for I am gentle and lowly in heart, and you will find rest for your souls. For my yoke is easy, and my burden is light." If you are off the track and know you need help, then get very still and listen carefully. You just may hear that still, small, quiet voice of God saying, *Come to Me. Come into My presence.*

Jesus was raised in the home of a carpenter. Carpenters didn't frame houses as they do today. They fashioned yokes and doors, which Jesus spoke of metaphorically. Picture two oxen yoked together pulling a heavy load. If only one is in the yoke, it is an encumbrance rather than a benefit. A yoke is only beneficial if two are in it and pulling together. Animal trainers will harness a young horse or an ox with an older, trained animal that has learned obedience. It was even said of Jesus, "Although he was a son, he learned obedience through what he suffered" (Hebrews 5:8).

The young ox may think the old ox is going too slow, and try to run on ahead, but they will only get a sore neck. Those who are inclined to burn the candle at both ends should listen to the words of Isaiah 40:28–31:

> Have you not known? Have you not heard? The Lord is the everlasting God, the Creator of the ends of the earth. He does not faint or grow weary; his understanding is unsearchable. He gives power to the faint, and to him who has no might he increases strength. Even youths shall faint and be weary, and young men shall fall exhausted; but they who wait for the Lord shall renew their strength; they shall mount up with wings like eagles; they shall run and not be weary; they shall walk and not faint.

Some just drop out and life becomes a drag, because the old ox will just keep on walking. Life goes on no matter what we do. Others will be tempted to stray off to the left or to the right, but the old ox just keeps a steady pace with his eyes on a sure destination. Some will throw off the yoke, because they want to live their own way at their own pace – to be their own lord and master. A wise young ox will begin to think, *This old ox knows how to walk and he knows where he is going. I think I will learn from him.* Those who do will learn to take one day at a time. They will learn the priority of relationships. They will learn to walk humbly with their God.

The context for this invitation to come to His presence is telling. Jesus had denounced "the cities where most of his mighty works had been done, because they did not repent" (Matthew 11:20). "At that time Jesus declared, 'I thank you, Father, Lord of heaven and earth, that you have hidden these things from the wise and understanding and revealed them to children; yes, Father, for such was your gracious will'" (verses 25–26). Jesus had previously warned His disciples about the problem of pride when He said, "Truly, I say to you, unless you turn and become like children, you will never enter the kingdom of heaven. Whoever humbles himself like this child is the greatest in the kingdom of heaven" (Matthew 18:3–4). Little children willingly believe what a loving parent tells them.

One of the surest ways to not experience the presence of God is to let our understanding determine our faith. After telling his readers that they had become partakers of God's divine nature, the apostle Peter wrote, "For this very reason, make every effort to supplement your faith with virtue, and virtue with knowledge, and knowledge with self-control, and self-control with steadfastness, and steadfastness with godliness, and godliness with brotherly affection, and brotherly affection with love" (2 Peter 1:5–7).

Faith is the foundation. We are saved by faith. We are sanctified by faith, and we live by faith. Virtue is built upon faith, and knowledge is built upon virtue. A child may say, "I don't understand why I have to do that," and the good parent says, "Because I told you to do it." It may be appropriate to explain later, but submission is the issue of the moment. Trust and obey and you will gain understanding. Do the right thing now and you will know why later. Much of the Western church has turned that around to our detriment. We want to fully understand before we choose to believe. Theologian and author Christopher Hall explains:

A primary dictum of the Western theological tradition, channeled through the conduit of Augustine and Anselm, had been that faith led to understanding. This was a faith in Christ grounded in personal self-awareness of sin and cognizant of the continual lure of self-deception, rooted in the intrinsic authority of Scripture and divinely inspired revelation it communicated, and nurtured by the church's history of reflection on the meaning of God's word to humanity.

The enlightenment perspective stood this approach on its head. Understanding would lead to a mature faith, rather than the reverse. Hence, those aspects of the Christian tradition that failed to meet the standards of human reason – liberated, autonomous reason – were regarded with suspicion and for many ultimately discarded. Is it surprising that the resurrection, incarnation, Trinity, miracles and other revelatory gifts became negotiables?[4]

If we believe only that which we can understand, we end up trusting ourselves and questioning God. "Does the clay say to him who forms it, 'What are you making?'" (Isaiah 45:9). Thinking we know better than God what is best for our lives is the audacity of arrogance. "For the foolishness of God is wiser than men, and the weakness of God is stronger than men" (1 Corinthians 1:25). It is childlike faith to "Trust in

---

4   Christopher Hall, *Reading Scripture with the Church Fathers* (Downers Grove, IL: Intervarsity Press, 1998), pp. 24–25

the Lord with all your heart, and do not lean on your own understanding. In all your ways acknowledge him, and he will make straight your paths" (Proverbs 3:5–6).

Another trick of the mind that keeps us from experiencing the presence of God is to search for an experience to validate truth. For instance, "We know that our old self was crucified with him [Jesus] in order that the body of sin might be brought to nothing, so that we would no longer be enslaved to sin" (Romans 6:6). I have been crucified with Christ. "It is no longer I who live, but Christ who lives in me" (Galatians 2:20). Many who struggle with understanding and appropriating such verses about who they are in Christ wonder, *What experience must I have in order for that to be true?* The only experience that had to happen in order for that to be true happened 2,000 years ago, and the only way we can appropriate that is by faith. We cannot do for ourselves what Christ has already done for us.

When I first get up in the morning (before coffee), I may feel alive to sin and dead to Christ. If I live that day believing what I feel, I will have a very bad day. Instead I get up in the morning and thank God for a new day. I choose to believe that I am alive in Christ and dead to sin, and when I live that day believing what God said is true, it works out in my experience. It isn't what we do that determines who we are; who we are determines what we do. So who are we?

See what kind of love the Father has given to us, that we should be called children of God; and so we are. The reason why the world does not know us is that it did not know him. Beloved, we are God's children now, and what we will be has not yet appeared; but we know that when he appears we shall be like him, because we shall see him as he is. And everyone who thus hopes in him purifies himself as he is pure. (1 John 3:1–3)

So how do we live in the presence of God and find rest for our souls? According to Jesus there is only one way: "The time is fulfilled, and the kingdom of God is at hand; repent and believe in the gospel" (Mark 1:15). The repentance process begins with salvation. Therefore, "Examine yourselves, to see whether you are in the faith. Test yourselves. Or do you not realize this about yourselves, that Jesus Christ is in you? – unless indeed you fail to meet the test!" (2 Corinthians 13:5). Christ in you is the hope for glory. Hope is the present assurance of some future good, and that good is the manifestation of God in your life. God is the One who grants repentance, which we can't do without Him. Repentance is God's means of resolving personal and spiritual conflicts.[5] This requires submitting to God and resisting the devil (James 4:7), who "prowls around like a roaring lion, seeking someone to devour" (1 Peter 5:8). In the earlier church there was a definitive process of becoming a communicant. Candidates would literally face the west and say, "I renounce you, Satan, and all your works, and all your ways." They would then face the east and make their profession of faith in God. Repentance removes the barriers to our intimacy with God, and it sets us free from our past. Human history flows from creation and freedom to the fall and bondage to sin, to redemption, to repentance and freedom. "For freedom Christ has set us free" (Galatians 5:1).

Living in the presence of God is the lifestyle of a true worshipper. Jesus told the woman at the well that where you worship God isn't the issue. He said that "the hour is coming, and is now here, when the true worshipers will worship the Father in spirit and truth, for the Father is seeking such people to

---

5   The purpose of Freedom in Christ Ministries is to equip the church worldwide, enabling it to establish its people, marriages, and ministries alive and free in Christ through genuine repentance and faith in God. The tool that we use to accomplish this is "The Steps to Freedom in Christ." Our ministry also has "Steps to Setting Your Marriage Free" and "Steps to Setting Your Church Free" for corporate conflict resolution.

worship him" (John 4:23). We worship God when we ascribe to Him His divine attributes, which should always be on our minds whenever and wherever we are. God doesn't need us to tell Him who He is. He is completely secure within Himself. He wants us to always be mindful of His loving presence.

When worship becomes a lifestyle, we start to see evidence of His presence everywhere, because "The heavens declare the glory of God, and the sky above proclaims his handiwork" (Psalm 19:1). Modern science is just getting a glimpse of how immense the universe is. We are just a speck on this planet, and the earth is just a speck in a galaxy that is just a speck in the universe. How big is our God who is far greater than His creation? If you are wondering why God who is so majestic could even know or care about your existence, then consider David's words in Psalm 8:3–6:

When I look at your heavens, the work of your fingers, the moon and the stars, which you have set in place, what is man that you are mindful of him, and the son of man that you care for him? Yet you have made him a little lower than the heavenly beings and crowned him with glory and honor. You have given him dominion over the works of your hands; you have put all things under his feet.

Our heavenly Father is intimately involved with every one of His children. He is omniscient. He knows how many strands of hair we have on our heads. He knows the thoughts and intentions of our hearts, which means we can pray with our thoughts. God didn't just sit on His throne and watch us suffer down here. He sent Jesus to be one of us. "For we do not have a high priest who is unable to sympathize with our weaknesses, but one who in every respect has been tempted as we are, yet without sin. Let us then with confidence draw near to the throne of grace, that we may receive mercy and find grace to help in time of need" (Hebrews 4:15–16). "So we do not lose heart. Though our outer nature is wasting away, our inner nature is being renewed day by day. For this slight momentary affliction is preparing for us an eternal weight of glory beyond all comparison" (2 Corinthians 4:16–17).

God is omnipresent, so we choose to believe that wherever we are, God is present. That realization changed how I do ministry. Whether I'm discipling, counseling, teaching, or preaching I begin with the following prayer: *Lord, I acknowledge Your presence in my life and in this setting. I declare my dependency upon You, for apart from Christ I can do nothing. I ask You to fill me with Your Holy Spirit, and superintend my choice of words. I ask this in the wonderful name of Jesus my Lord and Savior.*

I'm sure the staff of our ministry has heard me pray that prayer many times and wondered if I will ever come up with something new to say. I have no problem being repetitious about something that is absolutely essential for the success of a mission. Jesus said, "My sheep hear my voice, and I know them, and they follow me" (John 10:27). I believe that, so I seek to be guided by Him. In all honesty I have gone on trips and realized that they were my idea and not God's. I have also come home from trips and said, "That was Your idea, wasn't it, God?" I believe that God is omniscient so I don't hesitate to ask Him for wisdom, "who gives generously to all without reproach" (James 1:5). I am still learning how not to lean on my own understanding, and when I catch myself doing so, I confess it to God. Confession means to agree with God, and is essentially the same as walking in the light. God's children don't need to ask His forgiveness every time they sin, because He has already forgiven all His children.

We practice the presence of God when we walk in the light, which means that we live in conscious moral agreement with God. We do so because "If we say we have fellowship with him while we walk in darkness, we lie and do not practice the truth. But if we walk in the light, as he is in the light, we have fellowship with one another, and the blood of Jesus cleanses us from all sin" (1 John 1:6–7). We can be completely honest with God, because we are already forgiven. He knows everything about us anyway, so why not be honest? That is so liberating and makes all our relationships honest and forthright. Living a lie is living in darkness.

I try not to usurp God's role, and I try to consider the other person more important than myself, which is to have the same mind as Christ (Philippians 2:3–5). When I struggle I draw near with confidence to the throne of grace that I may receive mercy and find grace to help in time of need (Hebrews 4:16). I'm anything but perfect, but I know God is with me, and I want to be with Him. We all have free choice, and I choose to believe God, and believe what He has revealed about Himself, and believing that has changed who I am and how I live.

Moses asked the right questions: who is going with me? Will You let me know Your ways? The answer is summed up in the Great Commission:

All authority in heaven and on earth has been given to me. Go therefore and make disciples of all nations, baptizing them in the name of the Father and of the Son and of the Holy Spirit, teaching them to observe all that I have commanded you. And behold, I am with you always, *to the end of the age (Matthew 28:18–20, emphasis added).*

6

Fully in His Presence

If sorrow, and mourning, and sighing and death itself assail us from the afflictions both of soul and body, how shall they be removed, except by cessation of their causes, that is to say, the afflictions of flesh and soul? Where will you find adversities in the presence of God? Where incursions of an enemy in the bosom of Christ? Where attacks of the devil in the face of the Holy Spirit – now that the devil himself and his angels are "cast into the lake of fire?" What plague awaits the redeemed from death after eternal pardon? What wrath is there for the reconciled after grace? What weakness after their renewed strength? What risk and danger after salvation?

Tertullian, *On the Resurrection of the Flesh*

I dropped by to see Joanne at noon today. I started off seeing her in the mornings and evenings, but as her struggle has progressed I have started coming back at noon. On this particular day I woke her up, and she said she had been having an exciting dream. At first I didn't pay much attention to what she said. One learns not to take too seriously what people with dementia are thinking and dreaming. She calls the nurse the librarian, or policeman, and pills are "the box," because they crush the pills, mix them with apple sauce, and serve them in a little container (box).

I helped her to the bathroom and did a lot of mini-preparations to get her settled for lunch. She asked me to turn on the television, which she never does. The television is more for me, and she prefers that the sound be muted. I have watched a few football games in silence. I said, "I don't need to watch anything, but tell me about the dream." She said, "It was exciting. I was in this parade in the desert with a host of Christians." It was so real to her that she wasn't sure she had been dreaming, which is why she asked me to turn on the TV. She wanted to see if it was in the news. "Was it peaceful?" I asked. "No, it was exciting!"

Joanne hasn't been excited about anything for a long time, and I sensed this was more than just a dream. The memory of the dream didn't fade like all her other short-term memories. I believe God is preparing her to come to be fully with Him. I have been talking to her about heaven, and what it will be like to be in God's presence. However, my words don't bring the same excitement. We can tell others that God loves them, but it doesn't have anywhere near the same impact as when they hear from God that He loves them. The same holds true for the conviction of sin. If I point out sins in others, they become defensive. If God points them out, they become convicted. I was filled with joy that God was speaking to my Babe, but what astonished me most was the timing. This morning she asked me, "Do people ever get well and leave this place?" I said, "Honey, there is only one known cure for what you are struggling with, and that is heaven." I have chosen to be honest with Joanne about her condition.

I had a similar visitation from God on my first trip to Israel, which was life changing. I was a pastor and was having a difficult time with a board member. I wasn't leading the tour, but I was the only pastor in the group. So I had the privilege to lead the communion service at the garden tomb, and baptize some folks in the Jordan River. That was inspirational, but the time I spent in the Garden of Gethsemane was life changing. The garden is at the base of the Mount of Olives, where one can see the Eastern Gate of the old walled city of Jerusalem. In the garden is a beautiful mosaic structure called the Church of All Nations that encompasses the rock where Jesus agonized in prayer. The day after we toured the garden I returned to the church by myself. I sat near the rock where Jesus contemplated what it meant to take all of the sins of the world upon Himself. He prayed, "Father, if you are willing, remove this cup from me. Nevertheless, not my will, but yours, be done" (Luke 22:42).

Head knowledge became heart knowledge that afternoon. Jesus had to take upon Himself all the sins of all the people of the world, and God was asking me to take the sins of one man upon myself. I thought, *I can do that. No! I will do that.* Forgiving others who don't deserve it is the most Christ-like thing we can do. A burden was lifted from me that day, and I felt lighter and freer than I had for some time.

When I had signed up for the tour I paid a little extra to have a private room. I didn't want to risk ruining the trip of a lifetime by having a snoring roommate, or worse. I went to sleep peacefully that night, but was awakened sometime in the middle of the night with an overwhelming sense of God's presence. There were no voices or visions. I felt like

I was suspended in time and space. All I could think was, *It's too good. It's too good. Is this what heaven is going to be like?* It lasted for some time, enough for me to know that it wasn't a dream. I awoke the next morning with the experience fresh in my memory. I have never forgotten it.

I had no idea at the time why God gave me a taste of His goodness, but I have no doubt then and now that it was God. In one sense nothing changed the next day. Life went on as usual. It was not a game changer in regards to my calling. I went home and continued being a husband, father, and pastor. However, I never once questioned the goodness of God from that day forward. In hindsight I think God knew there were some hard days ahead for us in ministry.[6] There have been some who have "meant evil against me, but God meant it for good" (Genesis 50:20). There is a price to pay for freedom. "Indeed, all who desire to live a godly life in Christ Jesus will be persecuted" (2 Timothy 3:12). We don't usually share that verse in our evangelistic meetings, but it sure is beneficial to know that God is good during those times.

"He [Jesus] is the radiance of the glory of God and the exact imprint of his nature, and he upholds

---

6   See my memoirs, *Rough Road to Freedom.*

the universe by the word of his power" (Hebrews 1:3). God is the ultimate reality. If He ceased to exist, so would everything else He created. He is everywhere present, but the non-believer doesn't know it. God is present with them, but they are not present with Him. God is also present with every believer, and we are partially present with Him. Asking God to be present with us is a subtle denial of His omnipresence. It is more appropriate to ask God to grant us a consciousness of His presence. It is best to believe that He is present and live accordingly by faith.

There are no perfect people, and our imperfections keep us from being fully present with God. We are privileged to get a taste of His glory now. It is just a sampling, but it is enough to keep us longing for our eternal home. We are not going to junk up heaven with our flesh patterns, decaying bodies, and partially renewed minds:

For we know in part and we prophesy in part, but when the perfect comes, the partial will pass away. When I was a child, I spoke like a child, I thought like a child, I reasoned like a child. When I became a man, I gave up childish ways. For now we see in a mirror dimly, but then face to face. Now I know in part; then I shall know fully, even as I have been fully known. (1 Corinthians 13:9–12)

I believe we need a resurrected body to be fully in the presence of God. Paul wrote:

> *There are heavenly bodies and there are earthly bodies, but the glory of the heavenly is of one kind, and the glory of the earthly is of another... So is it with the resurrection of the dead. What is sown is perishable; what is raised is imperishable. It is sown in dishonor; it is raised in glory. It is sown in weakness; it is raised in power. It is sown a natural body; it is raised a spiritual body. (1 Corinthians 15:40, 42–44)*

Jesus was with us in a natural body with all its physical limitations. His resurrected body was completely different, with one visible exception. "On the evening of that day, the first day of the week, the doors being locked where the disciples were for fear of the Jews, Jesus came and stood among them and said to them, 'Peace be with you.' When he had said this, he showed them his hands and his side" (John 20:19–20). There were no natural barriers for the resurrected Jesus. A locked door couldn't keep Him out. I believe that we shall someday see those imprints on His side and feet, and it will serve as an eternal reminder of the cost of our rebellion.

When I was a pastor a couple joined our church,

but only the wife attended Sunday morning. Emerson was confined to his home because of emphysema. He needed an oxygen bottle to stay alive. I visited him several times, and he talked of past glories. He had played minor league baseball and played the harmonica, which I do as well. He gave me his collection, because he no longer had the lungs to play them. One was a base harmonica, which I had never seen before. He took a turn for the worse and ended up in the hospital. I stopped by every day, but one Saturday afternoon his wife called, and said, "Emerson has given up. Can you go see him tonight and encourage him to keep fighting?"

I did go to see him, but I called his wife after I returned home. I said, "I think we are doing the wrong thing. Emerson has no will to live and we are making him feel guilty. I think we should let him die a peaceful natural death. With your permission I would like to stop by the hospital tomorrow morning before I go to church and tell him how good heaven is going to be. He'll zip around the bases and play his harmonica again."

There was a pause, and finally she said, "You're right. Yes, you have my permission."

The next morning I told him how good it was going to be in heaven, and that he would have a new resurrected body. After church I took my family to lunch, and when we got home the phone was ringing. A tearful, but grateful, wife said, "Emerson died late this morning in peace. Thank you for helping him make that transition."

Modern science has made it possible to artificially prolong our natural life, but that is not necessarily a blessing. The ultimate value is not our natural life; it is our spiritual life in Christ, which we will not lose when we physically die. Actually we will experience an incredible gain by being fully in the presence of God. Paul said, "For to me to live is Christ, and to die is gain" (Philippians 1:21). That is not a license to commit suicide, because we are called to be good stewards of the life He has entrusted to us. However, the person who is free from the fear of death is free to live today. I have no desire to prolong Joanne's suffering. I just want her to die in dignity, so she can enjoy her reward. My goal is to make that transition as pleasant as possible and patiently await God's timing. We should seek His presence now, and look forward to being fully in His presence when He calls us home.

Jesus said, "Let not your hearts be troubled. Believe in God; believe also in me. In my Father's house are many rooms. If it were not so, would I have told you that I go to prepare a place for you? And if

I go and prepare a place for you, I will come again and will take you to myself, that where I am you may also be" (John 14:1–3). I believe heaven is a prepared place, but I don't think of it in the same way that I do the three-dimensional world that I presently relate to with my natural senses. Even in our present state the only sanctuary we have is our position in Christ:

> God, being rich in mercy, because of the great love with which he loved us, even when we were dead in our trespasses, made us alive together with Christ — by grace you have been saved — and raised us up with him and seated us with him in the heavenly places in Christ Jesus, so that in the coming ages he might show the immeasurable riches of his grace in kindness toward us in Christ Jesus. (Ephesians 2:4–7)

The present position we already have in Christ is "far above all rule and authority and power and dominion, and above every name that is named, not only in this age, but also in the one to come. And he put all things under his feet and gave him as head over all things to be the church, which is his body, the fullness of him who fills all in all" (Ephesians 1:21–23). We may not fully understand what it means to be seated with Christ in the heavenlies, but we don't have to understand in order to believe. I choose to believe that God has forgiven me, given me new life in Christ, and seated me with Christ in heavenly places, which is far above all rule and authority. Satan has no authority over me, or any of God's children. He can't do anything about our position in Christ, but if he can persuade us to believe it isn't true, we will live as though it isn't.

Jesus has all authority in heaven and on earth and He has commissioned us to make disciples of all nations. Our message is simple. Believe in the Lord Jesus Christ and you shall be saved. There is a hell to be avoided and a heaven to be gained. Until then all of creation is groaning and awaiting the final redemption. The apostle Paul puts it in perspective in Romans 8:18–24:

> *For I consider that the sufferings of this present time are not worth comparing with the glory that is to be revealed to us. For the creation waits with eager longing for the revealing of the sons of God. For the creation was subjected to futility, not willingly, but because of him who subjected it, in hope that the creation itself will be set free from its bondage to decay and obtain the freedom of the glory of the children of God. For we know that the whole creation has been groaning together in the pains of childbirth until now. And not only creation, but*

we ourselves, who have the firstfruits of the Spirit,
groan inwardly as we wait eagerly for adoption as
sons, the redemption of our bodies. For in this hope
we were saved.

There is a new earth and a new heaven coming. There is no way that we can humanly imagine what it will be like to be in the presence of eternal good, where all evil has been banished. Our resurrected bodies will experience no decay, physical pain or abnormalities. "Oh, taste and see that the Lord is good! Blessed is the man who takes refuge in him" (Psalm 34:8).

Many years ago I read a study about how different segments of society view death, which was conducted in the pre-civil rights era. Most of the Caucasian Christian community approached death with fear and trepidation. It was not something to look forward to. After all, could life be any better than playing golf at the Augusta National Country Club in 80 degree weather sipping a lemonade? If you have worked hard all your life to have heaven on earth, you probably haven't stored up many treasures in heaven. If you aim for this world, you just may miss the next. If you aim for the next world, you get the pleasure of His presence now and the hope of being fully in His presence in the new heaven and new earth.

It was just the opposite for the African American

Christian community. They were not experiencing heaven on earth, and they saw death as good, and not something to be feared. They were taught from the days of slavery to look forward to the Promised Land. Martin Luther King, Jr. introduced the idea that some of that Promised Land could be realized now.

When I was teaching at Talbot School of Theology, I was asked to be the speaker for an older adult Sunday School class. There were about forty couples in their sixties and seventies, and a few singles who had lost their spouses. I talked about preparing for impermanence, and how important it was to have plans in place should one of them die. Most had a will, but very little had been discussed beyond that. I was totally surprised. It is tragic to leave details about finances, funerals, and burial sites to the bereaved. It is just as tragic to not think through the issues of life before a crisis hits.

I had started a Bible study at work when I was an engineer, and I kept inviting an intern to come who was riding with me to work. Finally he said, "I'm just not interested in religion anymore. Okay?" Sensing something had turned him off, I asked if he would be willing to share what it was. He told me that he had been very involved in church years earlier, as was his older brother whom he idolized. One day his brother was killed in an automobile accident, and the next day his wife committed suicide. In deep grief he went to see the pastor. The intern said, "If that man had said nothing I probably would still be going to church, but I couldn't accept what he said." I am thankful to this day that I heard that before I went into ministry. In the middle of a crisis the wrong words can turn people off for all eternity. We would accomplish a lot more if we learned to say nothing and weep with those who weep.

The worldly think they have all the answers until it comes to death. The first time I did a funeral I stood at the head of the casket as the people filed by. I was totally surprised at my own discernment. I felt like I could say with certainty which ones were believers and which ones weren't. Both could be showing emotional stress, so it wasn't a psychological differentiation. It was truly spiritual. It had such a big impact on me that I asked another pastor if he had had such an experience. Physical death is the great divide for believers and unbelievers, and the greatest opportunity to share the love of Christ comes when death is imminent.

I was the college pastor in a large church and I was counseling a friend on a Tuesday afternoon when the telephone rang. One of my college students, Zandra Kelly, said, "Pastor Neil, my grandmother was supposed to die last Saturday night. They were going to stop all life support and the family had gathered to pay their final respects, but she didn't die. She is not a Christian and she may become conscious. Can you come to the hospital and see her?"

I invited the man in my office to come with me and he did. Zandra had told me that she and her mother would be there, and that they were the only two Christians in the entire family. I heard the labored breathing before we entered the room, but Zandra and her mother weren't there. My friend took one look and said, "I'll wait in the hall." The woman was lying at an odd angle on the bed and looked a pitiful sight. Her arms were blue with collapsed veins, and her eyes were crossed. I tried to communicate with her, but there was no response. *Lord, what do I do?* I wasn't expecting an answer, but immediately I had a distinct impression on my mind to sing to her. *Sing to her!* I was really thankful my friend had left the room.

I started to sing little choruses, not knowing what to expect. After a few minutes I saw her eyes uncross and she was looking at me. I introduced myself, and said I was there because Zandra had asked me to drop by. There was no response. "If you can hear me would you blink your eyes or raise your hands?" I asked. I was on her right side, but nothing moved. Then I saw her left hand lift slightly. So I walked around to the other side of the bed, and said again, "If you can hear me, raise your left hand." It came up slightly and she was looking at me. I said, "I'm here to tell you that God loves you. He loves you so much that He sent His only Son to die for all our sins and to give us new life." I never heard one spoken word from her during that whole time, but it just seemed like her lips pursed and she was asking, *Why?* So I explained the whole gospel and asked her, "Would you like to invite Jesus into your life? If so raise your left hand." It came up. I told her that God knew her thoughts, and she could make that decision in her mind. So I encouraged her to say a prayer with me, and I led her through a sinner's prayer where she indicated her choice to believe that Jesus died for her sins and came to give her eternal life.

Five minutes later Zandra came back to the room with her mother. They had gone to the cafeteria, and were surprised that I had already been there for half an hour. I met them at the door and said, "I need to prepare you for this. Your mother and grandmother just gave her heart to God. You are going to be a little surprised at what you see." They rushed by me and saw a newly born child of God smiling and looking at them with tears flowing down her face. I invited my friend to take another look, and he was shocked at the transformation. She lived for two more years and then went to be with her Father. I had changed churches during that time, but the family asked me to do the funeral. Probably all of the family had heard that story, and many came to Christ that day.

Now, I sit in silence with my wife of forty-nine years. I hear her groaning for the day of redemption. I have experienced the presence of God in her final months in ways that I never have before. Thank You, Jesus.

> *Blessed be the God and Father of our Lord Jesus Christ, the Father of mercies and God of all comfort, who comforts us in all our affliction, so that we may be able to comfort those who are in any affliction, with the comfort with which we ourselves are comforted by God. For as we share abundantly in Christ's sufferings, so through Christ we share abundantly in comfort too. (2 Corinthians 1:3–5)*

I hope I am in Joanne's presence when "morning comes." God has always been with her, and then Joanne will be fully with Him. She will be much better off than I am. I will miss her. She has been my wife and best friend for nearly fifty years. We have been through a lot together, and I am a much better person because Joanne said "I will" on June 4, 1966. When she is gone I will continue serving God until He calls me home. Until then I will help as many as I can find their identity and freedom in Christ so that they too may experience the presence of God who wants all His children to know the following:

You have been accepted.

John 1:12	You are God's child.
John 15:15	You are Jesus' friend.
Romans 5:1	You have been accepted (justified) by God.
1 Corinthians 6:17	You are united with the Lord and one with Him in spirit.
1 Corinthians 6:20	You have been bought with a price. You belong to God.
1 Corinthians 12:27	You are a member of Christ's body; you are part of His family.
Ephesians 1:1	You are a saint.
Ephesians 1:5	You have been adopted as God's child.
Ephesians 2:18	You have direct access to God through the Holy Spirit.
Colossians 1:14	You have been bought back (redeemed) and forgiven of all your sins.
Colossians 2:10	You are complete in Christ.

You are secure.

Romans 8:1–2	You are free from condemnation.
Romans 8:28	You are assured that all things work together for good.
Romans 8:31f	You are free from any condemning charges against you.
Romans 8:35f	You cannot be separated from the love of God.
2 Corinthians 1:21	You have been established, anointed, and sealed by God.
Colossians 3:3	You have died and your life is hidden with Christ in God.
Philippians 1:6	You can be sure that the good work that God has begun in you will be finished.
Philippians 3:20	You are a citizen of heaven.
2 Timothy 1:7	You have not been given a spirit of fear, but of power, love, and a sound mind.
Hebrews 4:16	You can find grace and mercy in time of need.
1 John 5:18	You are born of God and the evil one cannot touch you.

You are significant.

Matthew 5:13	You are the salt of the earth and light of the world.
John 15:1, 5	You are a part of the true vine, joined to Christ and able to produce much fruit.
John 15:16	You have been chosen by Jesus to bear fruit.
Acts 1:8	You are a personal witness of Christ's resurrection.
1 Corinthians 3:16	You are a temple of God.
2 Corinthians 5:17f	You have peace with God and are a minister of reconciliation.
2 Corinthians 6:1	You are God's co-worker.
Ephesians 2:6	You are seated with Christ in the heavenlies.
Ephesians 2:10	You are God's workmanship.
Ephesians 3:12	You may approach God with freedom and confidence.
Philippians 4:13	You can do all things through Christ who strengthens you.

Further Resources

All resources below written by Dr. Neil T. Anderson.

Core material

Victory Over the Darkness with study guide, audiobook, and DVD (Bethany House, 2000). With over 1,300,000 copies in print, this core book explains who we are in Christ, how to walk by faith in the power of the Holy Spirit, how to be transformed by the renewing of our mind, how to experience emotional freedom, and how to relate to one another in Christ.

The Bondage Breaker with study guide and audiobook (Harvest House Publishers, 2000), and DVD (Regal Books, 2006). With over 1,300,000 copies in print, this book explains spiritual warfare, what our protection is, ways that we are vulnerable, and how we can live a liberated life in Christ.

Breaking Through to Spiritual Maturity (Bethany House, 2000). This curriculum teaches the basic message of Freedom in Christ Ministries.

Discipleship Counseling with DVD (Bethany House, 2003). This book combines the concepts of discipleship and counseling, and teaches the practical integration of theology and psychology, for helping Christians resolve their personal and spiritual conflicts through repentance and faith in God.

Steps to Freedom in Christ and interactive video (Bethany House, 2004). This discipleship counseling tool helps Christians resolve their personal and spiritual conflicts through genuine repentance and faith in God.

Restored (E3 Resources). This book is an expansion of the *Steps to Freedom in Christ*, and offers more explanation and illustrations.

Walking in Freedom (Bethany House, 2008). This book is a twenty-one-day devotional that we use for follow-up after leading someone through the Steps to Freedom.

Freedom in Christ (Bethany House, 2008) is a discipleship course for Sunday School classes and small groups. The course comes with a teacher's guide, a student guide, and a DVD covering twelve lessons and the Steps to Freedom in Christ. This course is designed to enable new and stagnant believers to resolve personal and spiritual conflicts and be established alive and free in Christ.

The Bondage Breaker DVD Experience (Harvest House, 2011) is also a discipleship course for Sunday School classes and small groups. It is similar to the one above, but the lessons are fifteen minutes instead of thirty minutes.

The Victory Series (Bethany House, 2014; 2015). This is an eight-book discipleship course that helps participants become firmly rooted in Christ, grow in Christ, live in Christ, and overcome in Christ. The book titles are: *God's Story for You, Your New Identity, Your Foundation in Christ, Renewing Your Mind, Growing in Christ, Your Life in Christ, Your Authority in Christ,* and *Your Ultimate Victory in Christ.*

Specialized books

The Bondage Breaker: The Next Step (Harvest House, 2011). This book has several testimonies of people finding their freedom from all kinds of problems, with commentary by Dr. Anderson. It is an important learning tool for encouragers, and offers help for those who struggle.

Overcoming Addictive Behavior, with Mike Quarles (Bethany House, 2003). This book explores the path to addiction and how a Christian can overcome addictive behaviors.

Overcoming Depression, with Joanne Anderson (Bethany House, 2004). This book explores the nature of depression, which is a body, soul, and spirit problem, and presents a holistic answer for overcoming this "common cold" of mental illness.

Liberating Prayer (Harvest House Publishers, 2011). This book helps believers understand the confusion in their minds when it comes time to pray, and why listening in prayer may be more important than talking.

Daily in Christ, with Joanne Anderson (Harvest House Publishers, 2000). This popular daily devotional is also being used by thousands of Internet subscribers every day.

Who I Am in Christ (Bethany House, 2001). In thirty-six short chapters, this book describes who we are in Christ and how He meets our deepest needs.

Freedom from Addiction, with Mike and Julia Quarles (Bethany House, 1997). Using Mike's testimony, this book explains the nature of chemical addictions and how to overcome them in Christ.

One Day at a Time, with Mike and Julia Quarles (Bethany House, 2000). This devotional helps those who struggle with addictive behaviors and explains how to discover the grace of God on a daily basis.

Freedom from Fear, with Rich Miller (Harvest House Publishers, 1999). This book explains anxiety disorders and how to overcome them.

Setting Your Church Free, with Dr. Charles Mylander (Bethany House, 2006). This book offers guidelines and encouragement for resolving seemingly impossible corporate conflicts in the church and also provides leaders with a primary means for church growth – releasing the power of God in the church.

Setting Your Marriage Free, with Dr. Charles Mylander (Bethany House, 2006.) This book explains God's divine plan for marriage and the steps that couples can take to resolve their difficulties.

Christ Centered Therapy, with Dr. Terry and Julie Zuehlke (Zondervan Publishing House, 2000). A textbook explaining the practical integration of theology and psychology for professional counselors.

Getting Anger Under Control, with Rich Miller (Harvest House Publishers, 1999). This book explains the basis for anger and how to control it.

Breaking the Strongholds of Legalism, with Rich Miller and Paul Travis (Harvest House Publishers, 2003). An explanation of legalism and how to overcome it.

Winning the Battle Within (Harvest House, 2008). This book shares God's standards for sexual conduct, the path to sexual addiction, and how to overcome sexual strongholds.

Restoring Broken Relationships (Bethany House, 2016). God has given the church the ministry of reconciliation. This book explains what that ministry is and how relationships can be restored with God and others.

The Daily Discipler (Bethany House, 2005). This practical systematic theology is a culmination of all of Dr. Anderson's books, covering the major doctrines of the Christian faith and the problems Christians face. It is a five-day-per-week, one-year study that will thoroughly ground believers in their faith.

Becoming a Disciple-Making Church (Bethany House, 2016). This book is like a briefing for pastoral leaders, showing them how they can disciple people from bondage to freedom, from fruitless converts to disciples who can reproduce themselves.

Rough Road to Freedom (Monarch Books, 2013). Dr. Anderson's memoirs.

For more information or to purchase the above materials contact Freedom in Christ Ministries:

Canada
freedominchrist@sasktel.net
www.ficm.ca

United Kingdom
info@ficm.org.uk
www.ficm.org.uk

United States
info@ficm.org
www.ficm.org

International
www.ficminternational.org

If you enjoyed this book, you might also enjoy Neil Anderson's memoir:

ROUGH ROAD TO FREEDOM

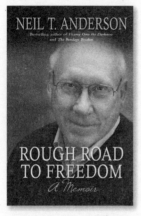

"This book is a jewel. We catch a glimpse of the man behind the movement, and praise God for the remarkable fruit."

– CHUCK MYLANDER, EFM DIRECTOR

Neil Anderson comes from a humble farming background. No one suspected that this fun-loving, athletic child would complete five degrees, author or co-author sixty books and found a global ministry. Neil served in the US Navy, then graduated in electrical engineering and worked as an aerospace engineer before sensing a call to ministry. He spent years as a church pastor and seminary professor before starting Freedom in Christ Ministries.

ISBN: 978 0 85721 294 8 | e-ISBN 978 0 85721 388 4

www.lionhudson.com

THE FREEDOM IN CHRIST DISCIPLESHIP COURSE

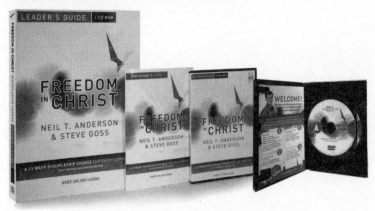

The Freedom In Christ Discipleship Course is an easy, effective way for any church to implement effective discipleship. Through 13 sessions, it helps Christians to resolve personal and spiritual conflicts through genuine repentance, so that they can take hold of the truth of who they are in Christ and move on to maturity.

For more information, or to find your local Freedom in Christ office, go to www.ficminternational.org

COURSE COMPONENTS

Leader's Guide	978-1-95424-939-5
Discipleship Course DVD Set	978-0-85721-665-6
Participant's Guide (single)	978-1-85424-940-1
Participant's Guide (pack of 5)	978-1-85424-941-8
Steps to Freedom in Christ DVD	978-1-85424-945-6
Steps to Freedom in Christ Participants Guide (single)	978-1-85424-943-2
Steps to Freedom in Christ Participants Guide (pack of 5)	978-1-85424-944-9